Shannon

Kathy McLaughlin

BACK TO LIFE

*One woman's inspiring triumph over
a series of terminal diagnoses*

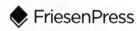 FriesenPress

Suite 300 - 990 Fort St
Victoria, BC, Canada, V8V 3K2
www.friesenpress.com

ISBN
978-1-4602-3489-1 (Hardcover)
978-1-4602-3490-7 (Paperback)
978-1-4602-3491-4 (eBook)

1. Biography & Autobiography, Medical

Distributed to the trade by The Ingram Book Company

Contents

DEDICATION

To Rob, Conor and Maddie, and my extended
family and treasured friends:

These moments we are sharing now are the moments I lived for.

My horoscope:

September 21, 1996

VIRGO (Aug. 23-Sept. 22): You can take care of legal, financial or medical issues with ease as long as you don't let uncertainty mess with your mind. Don't second-guess yourself about what you should do next. ★★★

We can't predict what will happen, we can only decide how we will be when things happen that are beyond our control. And when they look darkest, we can still find the light. We can triumph against all odds. I know, because this is my story... Kathy

3

Kathy McLaughlin is the rarest of people who, through her powerful intention and an alignment of miracles, has been released into the spiritual realm of life. I believe she has survived two supposedly hopeless medical situations so she can offer her great love, wisdom and inspiration to the world.

- Dr. Rob Rutledge, Radiation Oncologist, Associate Professor in the Faculty of Medicine at Dalhousie University & co-author, The Healing Circle

1

A CHANGE OF FLIGHT PLANS

Smooth cruising

It is my 40th birthday. It is a gorgeous September day, my favourite time of year. I arise full of potential, eagerly awaiting all that life has in store for me today and for the rest of my life. I have looked forward to this milestone, proud of what I have accomplished thus far, and with no reason to suspect that my destiny will not continue to unfold according to my plan.

I am on top of my game. I am happily married, we have two brilliant children, live in a big house in a wonderful neighbourhood with a fabulous view of Vancouver. I have an enviable position as vice president of western region with Rogers, a national wireless company. I live near my twin sister Carol, with whom I am very close, my brother Andy, my Mom, Dad and stepmom, Rob's parents and siblings. We have a strong network of good friends with whom we socialize regularly, enjoying tennis, skiing, bridge, golf and curling on a regular basis. I realize I live a charmed existence, but I believe I have earned this. I work hard – very hard – and have one of the toughest jobs of any woman I know. Underneath the surface, I suppress pangs of guilt – or perhaps regret – that I work such long hours and travel so frequently that I cannot spend as much time as

I would like with Rob, Conor and Maddie. At six and four, the kids are well cared for by our nanny and Rob is always home at night when I am not, so it is a sacrifice I make to continue to earn at the level that allows us to enjoy this lifestyle. I don't think of it as a life-threatening sacrifice, nor a soul-wrenching one, perhaps because I don't stop to really think about it.

Rob is up when I arise, and greets me cheerily with his usual birthday taunt, "What day is it?" accompanied by a cackle. I get a big smooch and then he's out the door as usual at 6:00 a.m. to be at his desk for the early morning market. He is at the peak of his career as a successful investment advisor. At this stage of our lives, we are confident that our financial future is assured as long as we continue to pay off the mortgage and stockpile for the kids' future education and our retirement.

I arrive at work to an office chock-full of balloons. Obviously, someone has tipped off my employees that it is a big birthday for me, as this is a highly unusual spectacle. I suspect Astrid, the proficient and motherly assistant I inherited along with the big office and big title, when my former boss vacated and left me in charge. Astrid has outlived two of my predecessors, but I am hoping not to fall prey to the revolving door.

That evening, Rob picks me up at work to depart for a surprise weekend on Saltspring Island. We indulge in a rare and romantic few days of idyllic relaxation. Rob has truly thought of everything, and I feel pampered and very special. I think how lucky I am to have him, and to still feel this way about each other after thirteen years of marriage.

All is well with the world.

Signs of turbulence

It is four months after my 40th birthday. I have found a lump on the left side of my neck, above my collar bone, nestled right next to my windpipe. A few weeks ago, I noticed a funny tight feeling in my throat. I poked around trying to identify the cause, and felt a small, soft tissue mass that moved underneath the skin. At the time I thought it might be a swollen gland from the nasty virus I was fighting, or perhaps a muscle pull from ferrying the kids up the rope tow on our ski holiday. In the busy happy time of the Christmas holidays, it had been quite easy to dismiss the possibility that it might be something else.

But now it is a Saturday morning in January, a cold, steely grey day, and I am in the bathroom, looking at myself in the mirror. I can no longer ignore this persistent intruder. I have to deal with the reality that it seems more like a lump than a sore muscle. But I am not one to tie up the medical system for non life-threatening ailments and I am wrestling with my inner parent who tells me I'm being overly paranoid. "Don't be silly," she says (she says that a lot…). "It's nothing. It's just a swollen gland from your flu." But there is that other, quieter inner voice urging me to make an appointment.

I go to the kitchen and make the call. The GP's office can fit me in on Monday, but I put them off until the following weekend. I always feel guilty about taking time off work for personal appointments, and I have a busy week ahead, including a trip to Montreal.

I am able to banish the lump to a background thought for the rest of the week, caught up in the frenetic imperatives of my business trip: back-to-back meetings, conference calls, presentations and business dinners.

On Saturday morning, I leave Rob in charge of the kids and breakfast dishes and duck out of the house, already ten minutes late for the doctor. I am annoyed with myself for making the appointment in the first place, thinking this will be an annoying waste of both my time and the doctor's. I am really wishing I was still lingering in the cozy warmness of Saturday morning at home.

Finally I am ushered in. I don the backless paper gown, suddenly feeling naked and vulnerable. The doctor breezes in, an imposing man at six foot two, but a kindly, fatherly sort. He asks the usual questions, pokes and prods the lump and the area around my windpipe, and then starts to look concerned. My stomach churns as I realize he is not going to brush this off as a minor ailment. "It is an enlarged lymph node," he explains. He then sucker punches me right in the queasy stomach by suggesting a biopsy. I am so rattled I laugh. I cannot fathom that he has any rational grounds for suggesting something so drastic for something I expected to be so trivial.

I ask him point-blank what he thinks it is.

"Well," he says, frowning, "the lymph node is inflamed. It could just be aggravated from some kind of infection in the respiratory tract. You did have a virus. But it could also indicate other conditions, including tuberculosis or lymphoma. It's best to have it biopsied right away, rather than wait."

I have no idea what lymphoma is, and am afraid to ask. Reading my mind, he clarifies that it is a form of cancer. I am trying to absorb this while waiting desperately for some final, reassuring words from the wise doctor. But he does not offer me the false hope of promising that it could be nothing. He recommends a surgeon who is usually available on short notice. *Shit*, I think. *This sounds serious.*

I leave the doctor's office with a referral in my pocket and a kindly pat on my shoulder – a compassionate gesture that only serves to heighten the level of my anxiety. I hustle to the car, jump in and start the motor before allowing myself to dissolve into tears. Fittingly, it is now raining. The rain trickles down the windshield in sympathy with my tears.

What now? Should I worry? I feel so helpless. How many countless patients have been through this vague diagnosis, the worry and the waiting? What did he say ... what did he say and why can't I remember anything after he said the word 'cancer'?

I drive home from the clinic alone with my racing thoughts and struggle to compose myself before entering the house. I find the kids happily playing in the family room with Laden, our live-in nanny, though she doesn't usually work on Saturdays. I am relieved to see her, having felt guilty about leaving Rob and the kids on a

Saturday morning, but I am jealous of her cheerful and carefree enjoyment of my children when I am exhausted from my trip and now stressed out from my visit to the doctor.

I put on a cheerful face, greet Conor and Maddie with a happy "Hello, Sweetnesses!" and then walk calmly through the house looking for Rob. I find him in the bathroom and can no longer maintain my composure. Erupting with the one emotion that seems available to me, I angrily blurt out the highlights of my visit to the doctor's office. "I have to go for a *biopsy*, for heaven's sake. Who's got time for *that*?!" After Rob gets over the initial surprise of my ambush, he lets me rant for a bit, and then taps the reservoir of patient strength he will draw on time and time again through the journey ahead. "Don't worry yet. Let's just wait and see."

Living on standby

Waiting is not my forte, and I know I will find it excruciatingly difficult to act as if everything is normal for the rest of the weekend. We agree not to say anything to anyone until we know for sure there is cause for concern.

Late on Sunday I remove the cone of silence and call Mom to tell her the news. Like Rob, she reassures me and promises not to worry, a promise I know she will not be able to keep despite her lifelong ability to maintain the appearance of upbeat optimism. Mom promises to pray, send pink light, invoke angels and summon her spirit guides. I do not argue, figuring I need all the help I can get.

Finally the weekend is over. Eager to get back to my work routine to get my mind off things, I leave before the kids are up. A month previously I had left my job at Rogers to start a new challenge as regional VP for Fido, a national telecommunications company launching a new wireless service across Canada. It is a fabulous opportunity, and I am enjoying it immensely despite the grueling schedule and daunting challenges of start-up. My days begin as early as 5:30 a.m. for eastern-time conference calls, and end well after 6 p.m., or later if we have evening training sessions or late supplier meetings.

Today, I have a long day ahead of me. I sit through the usual four-hour Monday morning conference call, but find it excruciatingly hard to focus. Afterwards, a Toronto colleague sends me a message: "You were pretty quiet today. Everything okay?" Gee, am I that transparent even on the *phone*?

"Wild weekend!☺" I text back, not wanting to get into it.

My evening is equally stressful. I have to chair a meeting with twenty blue-suited lawyers, accountants and other board members of a local theatre company.

As the meeting approaches I pull out the board package, but have no appetite for the cramming required to be moderately well briefed on the various agenda items. I have all the reasons in the world to beg off and ask another board member to stand in for me. But I cannot give myself permission to renege on such a serious commitment. It is not in my playbook to "call in sick", especially when I am not really sure I *am* sick. So I slog through the package, fighting off more than the usual level of pre-meeting jitters. By the time I enter the boardroom I am feeling slightly panicky and fighting a pounding headache. I put on my game face, greet the Board and go stiffly through the motions – literally and figuratively. At last it's over. I arrive home just after 10 p.m., exhausted and worried. Once again, Rob and the kids are already asleep. My appointment with the surgeon is tomorrow.

I arrive at the appointment early, eagerly hoping the surgeon will provide some answers. But this unfamiliar doctor is inscrutable, unemotional and noncommittal. He asks me all of the matter-of-fact history questions but will not speculate on what the lump might represent. He says the procedure will consist of full surgery under a general anesthetic, rather than a needle aspiration. I did not know an aspiration was a possible option, but this doctor states everything in a manner that implies I already know what is going on, discouraging questions. He adds to my alarm when he says that the surgery will be classified as urgent, and he will have a pathologist in attendance. "We'll see," is all he says when I press for his suspicions.

He advises me that his office will call me when they have a surgery date. Normally I find myself assertively negotiating with doctors, dentists, teachers and others to rearrange personal appointments to accommodate my work commitments. This will not be one of those times.

For the rest of the week I try to relegate this medical interruption to the role of a minor annoyance. I focus on my work routines and the rhythm of family life, with Rob as my co-conspirator in pretending everything is normal. On Sunday morning I pack and get ready to fly for my business trip. I cannot deny the sinking feeling in the pit of my stomach. Leaving Rob and the kids for these trips is always difficult, but this time I find myself on the verge of tears. Conor and Maddie are happily watching a Disney video with Laden, trusting that I will return as usual and life will be as it always is. I know these frequent trips take a toll on me, tearing a little hole in my heart each time I walk out the door and jump in the taxi. My little ritual is to sing a hammed-up version of "The Taxi Song" to the kids before I leave, but this time I can't get past the words "the taxi's waiting, he's blowing his horn ..." without choking up. Usually, I get all the way through "already I'm so lonesome I could cry". The kids don't seem to notice my warbly voice, so I smile bravely, peck everyone on the cheek and run up the driveway to the waiting cab.

This trip is mercifully short. We meet with the advertising agency to review creative concepts for the launch campaign. I enjoy having input to the marketing approach and the head office team welcomes my feedback on the proposed campaign. It helps me to get my mind off my personal worries.

Destination unknown

It is only during the plane trip home that I finally allow myself the luxury of really thinking about my health situation. I often use these five-hour flights for thinking time. I like the metaphor of being removed from terrestrial reality, floating above the clouds in suspended animation while the world scurries about its business below. I always arrive at my destination with renewed conviction about my life direction– an update of my flight plan, so to speak.

This time, I try to visualize a positive outcome from the biopsy – that the doctors will find the lump is benign. As I reflect on what is to come, I notice a strangely positive feeling of anticipation that alleviates some of the fear I feel about the possible diagnosis. As I analyze the source of this feeling, I realize that it stems from the sense of relief I have enjoyed during previous short hospital visits for minor surgery – for a tonsillectomy, rhinoplasty and of course for Conor and Maddie's births. My mom once commented on her delight in having the quiet, uninterrupted luxury of her hospital time when my brother Andy was born. There is something therapeutic and de-stressing about knowing you are not in charge; that someone else is attending to things. It is a moment of respite from the treadmill; a luxury I have not learned to grant myself without an excuse.

But in any of my previous hospital stays, I had a great deal of confidence in the outcome. This time it's different. I am wrestling with fear and uncertainty, the possibility of not being cured. I reflect on what a cancer diagnosis might mean. I have arrived at this stage of mid-life with a personal belief that illness is not completely arbitrary. I don't exactly believe that one causes one's own illness, but I think perhaps each illness contains a message, a clue about possible sources of discord in your life, alias "dis-ease". What if I do have cancer? What messages might my body be signaling? I jot down the first possibilities that come to mind:

If I have cancer, what is my body trying to tell me?

- *I have been ignoring my physical wellness in favour of work*
- *I have been ignoring myself in favour of work*
- *I have been burning myself out with overtime, frequent travel, overeating, drinking, late night office social parties, and a punishing work pace*
- *I am living with internal stress, fear of being proven incompetent, fear of failure*
- *I need more time with my family, with Rob, Conor and Maddie, Mom and Dad, my sister, brother, friends*
- *I need to reassess my life's priorities*
- *My soul is trying to get my attention*

As with any other challenge I have faced to this point in my life, I work away at generating possible theories to identify the most likely "root cause", so I can come up with strategies and action plans to fix the problem. It is my version of soul searching, but I recognize that I am still operating at a self-protective distance from soul work, more like a corporate project manager searching for solutions. Applying my business-trained analytical skills seems to help me process the situation.

Strangely, I find I am not questioning if the cancer is real. It doesn't seem to matter. The message is valid, regardless. And, despite the noncommittal responses from my surgeon, I realize that deep down I already believe it is cancer. My response is almost one of resignation to something I have seen coming and should have nipped in the bud much earlier. I know I have allowed myself to get run down, to get depleted physically, emotionally and spiritually. I realize that the questions I need to face relate to why I have allowed that to happen. It will take longer than a plane trip to find the answers.

2

At Least it's Trendy

A week after the surgery, I am ushered into the examining room.

"Well," says the surgeon, "it's as we suspected. You have Hodgkin's Disease."

"What?" I blurt out loud, wondering silently, *As who suspected?* I have no idea what Hodgkin's Disease is, and I certainly didn't suspect it.

"What-is-Hodgkin's-Disease?" I manage to emit slowly, as if speaking to an idiot. "Is it hereditary?" Somehow in my confused state I had jumped to the supposition that diseases with their own surnames must be genetic.

"No," he says, "it's not. It's the disease Mario Lemieux had." As if that explains everything. Despite my lifelong disinterest in Canada's national sport, I seem to recall that Lemieux is, or was, a famous hockey player. "Oh," I manage, and smile weakly, impressed that I have remembered this, and also that I have something famous. "At least it's trendy." We laugh, and he seems relieved and surprised not to have to be consoling the newly-diagnosed cancer patient. Why am *I* trying to make *him* feel better?

"But we are talking about ... cancer ... right?" I clarify, immediately extinguishing the effects of our brief moment of levity.

"Yes," he says. He goes on to describe Hodgkin's lymphoma as a cancer of the lymphatic system that has an eighty to ninety per cent cure rate when diagnosed early. He believes mine has been caught at an early stage, but he will refer me to an oncologist to properly stage the disease and decide on treatment.

"If you're going to get cancer, this is the one to get," he says.

He refers me to an oncologist who, he says, will call me soon. That's it. He takes off his white coat and goes to put his jacket back on, signifying that our transaction is completed. "Thank you," I say.

Rob has not even arrived by the time I am dismissed. The appointment, from my arrival to the abrupt pronouncement of my potentially terminal illness, has taken about fifteen minutes. I encounter Rob in the ground floor lobby as I am getting off the elevator. "Done already?" he says cheerfully. Then he reads my face, diagnosing the bewildered frown.

"I-have-Hodgkin's-Disease" I blurt for the first of many thousands of times to come. "Eighty to ninety per cent cure rate ... Mario Lemieux ... if you're going to get cancer, this is the one to get," stumbling through a patter I will later perfect.

We kiss and then drive convoy-style home. I pull into the driveway. No sign of Rob. Absurdly, I wonder if he has crashed behind me and I never noticed because of my cancer fog. But then I conclude, logically, that husbands just *don't* crash their cars 10 minutes after their wives have been diagnosed with cancer ... it just doesn't happen that way. And then he pulls into the driveway. We walk into the house together, opening the door to the new reality of our lives with cancer.

Pick your poison

From that day in March 1997, I was quickly swept up in a surprisingly efficient system that seems to suddenly fire on all cylinders when the patient is potentially terminal. My oncologist was a very efficient, matter of fact, experienced professional. He seemed quite certain about my treatment, the outcome and the side effects.

But an element of uncertainty was introduced when I was asked to participate in a clinical trial offering two alternate courses of treatment. My oncologist seemed unimpressed with the whole procedure as it involved a random draw and he strongly favoured one of the two courses of treatment – the more experimental one. It involved more aggressive chemotherapy for a shorter period, and no radiation. In Canada, at that time, the second treatment was more traditional, using a milder form of chemotherapy combined with radiation. My doctor's concern was that the radiation had been shown to cause other forms of cancer later in life; hence his preference for me was the aggressive chemotherapy. However, he cautioned, the chemotherapy was quite toxic and could cause side effects that were potentially fatal unless it was well monitored by doctor and patient.

To confirm my diagnosis and get another opinion on the recommended treatment, he sent me to a "cancer conference" at the BC Cancer Agency. The head of the team was a North American authority on lymphoma.

The conference panelists confirmed my doctor's diagnosis, but recommended the conservative treatment including radiation. To complicate things, that was also the treatment I drew for the clinical trial. Many people might have surrendered to the conventional consensus at this stage, but I was not satisfied because my oncologist had planted seeds of doubt about the long term side effects of the conservative treatment. Even though he was prepared to defer to the consensus, I was not. I asked him if I could get a *third* opinion, from a celebrated local oncologist whom many friends and neighbours had recommended. He agreed, though it was somewhat unconventional to get a third opinion. For me, it was the only way of obtaining reassurance.

The third doctor's opinion was to opt for the aggressive chemotherapy-only treatment. This oncologist explained that I was just too young to take the risk of having bladder or organ cancer later in life as a possible by-product of the radiation. "If you were twenty years older, perhaps, but we want you to have a good long life," he said, with a kindly pat on the shoulder. I was consumed by gratitude for this compassionate man.

It was decided: I was to commence four rounds (eight treatments) of aggressive chemotherapy in two weeks; less than a month after my surgery, and just two months from my decision to go to the doctor about my lump. It had all happened so quickly that I still felt like I might wake up the next morning and life would be back to normal.

Letting the C-word out of the bag

Rob and I decided to tell everyone what was going on now that we had the diagnosis and treatment plan. With the exception of my mom, sister and a few close friends, no one really knew what we had been going through. Of course we had advised Laden. Now it was time to have a quiet little sit-down with Conor and Maddie. At five and nearly seven, they were a little young to understand the full meaning of "Mommy's going to be sick for a while." I tried to keep things light-hearted, just saying I had a sickness that would mean I had to have some treatments and would need to rest a lot afterwards. I also let them know that it was highly likely that my hair would all fall out. Conor laughed at the thought of a bald mom, but Maddie cried, which made me cry too.

Coming out of the closet about my cancer opened an unexpected floodgate of compassion. The reaction of family, friends, neighbours and business colleagues to my news was immediate and overwhelming. I had no idea the extent to which people would find it in their hearts to reach out to me with cards, flowers, phone calls, emails, handwritten notes, books, poems, drop-in visits, care packages and baked goods.

I turned to the tough task of advising my employer of my situation. I called my boss, Jacques, in Montreal and told him the story. He was amazingly compassionate. He told me they would do whatever I needed to support me through this. I wanted to continue working and just take time off for my treatments as needed. He immediately reassured me that the company would pay my full salary for any of the time I needed to take off. Once again, I was deeply moved. This kind man showed a degree of emotion and support that I had never really experienced in a work setting. It was another in a series of little epiphanies to which cancer seemed to have opened the door.

I had only been in my job for three months; just long enough to hand pick a dream team of managers who shared with me the mandate of setting up a regional operation of Fido, a new mobile phone company. We had the minor assignment of hiring and training five hundred employees in the next three months to meet our launch date, while setting up all of the systems and processes needed to open our doors to customers. I had already hired fifty people, created the budget and business plan, signed leases for our store locations and assisted head office in developing the marketing and distribution plans for this new enterprise. I was having the time of my life. My eager young team had bought into the exciting vision of what we were creating. It was incredibly hard to suddenly have to advise them that I might not be a full participant in the journey.

I called the team together for what was one of the most difficult meetings of my life. We had a normal business planning meeting, and then at the end I said I had some news to share. I told them my story. Two of the six around the table started to cry, which didn't help me to maintain the positive tone and message that I had rehearsed. One of my managers later said my announcement was the bravest thing she had ever seen. I took a lot of pride in that statement. I wanted to be seen as brave. I didn't want to be seen as weak, vulnerable, sick, pitiable, scary, ghoulish, or any of those other things that members of the Cancer Club have to deal with in other peoples' reactions.

The bald truth

I commenced treatment the following week. My chemo appointments took about four hours every two weeks. I chose to have them on Friday afternoons so I could recuperate on the weekend and return to work on Mondays. The oncologist was certain I would lose all of my hair, but I hoped and prayed I would be one of the lucky ones who somehow escaped this telltale hallmark of the Club. I would notice some hair loss five weeks after the first treatment, he said, and then it would take about three days for all of it to go.

My long hair had always been a source of pride. I wore it tied up for work, in a French braid or roll, and enjoyed wearing it down or in a ponytail on weekends. I could not bear the thought of pulling out handfuls of my long locks. In defiance, I went to my hairdresser, told him everything and asked for his best work. He gave me a "news anchor haircut". After I got over the shock of the mountain of hair on the floor, we both agreed I looked like Diane Sawyer.

Maddie cried and ran out of the room when I came home with the new cut. Rob said all the appropriate nice things about how sexy I looked, and Conor smiled uncertainly, not sure which way to side.

I got rave reviews at work, but I thought they were all being polite – or worse, sympathetic – and I missed my hair terribly. It was hardest when I visited my sister Carol that weekend. Identical twins, we had generally sported similar hairstyles. It was like looking in the mirror and seeing my old hair, and it made me dread even more deeply the possibility that I would soon be bald.

Carol and I have always been as close as you would expect twin sisters to be. She knew instinctively that I was not comfortable with my "new look", and made an appointment to take me wig-shopping the following weekend. By the end of the week, right on schedule, my hair started to fall out in gentle little fingerfuls, thankfully not in clumps as I had expected. I met Carol at a wig shop in Chinatown for an afternoon of gay abandon trying on everything in the store. We laughed until we cried as I morphed into Conway Twitty, Dolly Parton, Marilyn Monroe and finally Alice Cooper. In the end, I bought a quite suitable synthetic "blonde bob" for two hundred dollars. I wore it home, feeling more like my former self.

Maddie had gotten used to me having less and less hair, but to help her process the reality of my impending baldness, I let her practice her hair design skills on my dwindling locks. She came up with a sporty really-short style that lasted about two days before my hair did finally come out in clumps. I remember it distinctly because it was the weekend Princess Diana met her sad demise. I watched the round-the-clock CNN coverage of the crash while pulling handfuls of hair from my head. Finally, I asked Rob to help me shave the rest with an electric leg razor – but quickly realized that is not a good idea. It left me with a scratchy, itchy stubble, which made wearing my wig quite uncomfortable.

I enjoyed my wig phase as it radically reduced my early morning prep-time, and I received many compliments on my "new do". I also enjoyed playing with hats, kerchiefs and turbans and the whole new world of head gear I'd never explored during my long hair rut.

One weekend I wore my wig to Maddie's soccer game. I usually wore it to the kids' activities because I knew they were both sensitive about having a "kerchief-mom" and all of the questions that begged, silent or otherwise. As I was settling in on the folding lawn chair I'd taken along to help with the chemo-fatigue, I spotted an old friend making a beeline towards me. As she approached, she shrieked, "Oh my gosh, I LOVE your new do! You really look fabulous! Where did you get it done?" Obviously, she had no idea it was a wig, and also had no idea that I had cancer. At first I didn't know what to say. But then I gently let her know I was battling lymphoma, at which point she was so horrified at her blunder she burst into tears. I tried to console her, and we dissolved into a big hug. Maddie glanced over from the field to see why we were carrying on, realized it was just another "cancer moment" and turned her attention back to the game.

3

THE ORIGINS OF DISEASE

Over the next few months, I got past the initial shock and worry of having cancer and settled into the routine of living as a cancer patient. I started to look forward to my treatments, as toxic as they were, because they represented welcome down-time for reading and continuing the soul-searching personal journey work I had started before being diagnosed. The chemo nurses were angels, saints, care-givers who really cared. There was a healing, therapeutic aura in the ward and I made the most of my days "off", using the time to try to understand why I had become sick and what psychological or spiritual stresses might have contributed. I wanted to try to isolate the point in time when I had become so compromised that I was a ready target for cancer, to avoid duplicating that set of conditions in the future.

I observed others in the chemo ward to see how they dealt with their disease and treatment. This ward was usually full, and one thing was clear – everyone was different. There was the elderly Iranian woman with leukemia, surrounded by daughters, talking up a storm in Farsi. There was the middle-aged mother with breast cancer, with her doting 20-something gay son. He listened patiently while she complained, apparently about financial concerns. He was kind and solicitous, without affectation, asking what she wanted to do when she got home and how he could make her more comfortable during the chemo side effects.

In the hospital library I found Dr. Bernie Siegel's *Love, Medicine & Miracles*. Dr. Siegel expresses the belief that chronic illness points to long term stressors that need to be healed, along with the illness, for one to make a whole recovery. His theory seems to be that the type of cancer you get contains a specific message about the source of the stress. He says to look for clues in something traumatic that happened in your life approximately eighteen months to two years prior to diagnosis.

Frances, the lady in the next chemo bed with the saintly son, was a member of the growing and significant Breast Cancer Club. I chatted with them about Dr. Siegel's theories, and both she and her son expressed the belief that breast cancer was about women learning to love themselves. "Breasts are our maternal, feminine, sexual, nurturing part," said Frances. "I believe my breast cancer is telling me to pay attention to my own needs instead of just nurturing everyone else."

But what about Hodgkin's Disease? My cancer originated in the lymph nodes in the chest area. The swollen lump I had first discovered had been pressing on my windpipe, causing an obstruction in my throat. I had laryngitis and at first had thought that was the cause of the swollen gland. Those who follow chakras say the throat region is the spiritual centre. Perhaps the cancer was signaling that I had suppressed my true voice.

The stress of success

There had been physical symptoms of stress-overload while I was in my previous job. Before accepting the start-up role with Fido, I had been the regional VP and General Manager of Rogers Wireless for western Canada. It had been a very difficult role for me, and by the time I was diagnosed, I had already escaped that job in favour of the exciting new role at Fido.

I scanned back over my last few years at Rogers to see if I could find some clues about the origins of my illness. I found many. In one instance I had an attack of nerves while leading a meeting that should have been well within my comfort zone. I was not alien to these attacks but over the years I had found ways of controlling my performance anxiety, and had become quite accomplished at speaking to groups. But this time I had been completely ambushed. As I launched into my introduction, I was overcome. I was unable to breathe, my voice was constricted, my heart was racing and I needed to run and hide. I could not disguise my symptoms – they were too prolonged and overt. I gasped and coughed, and mumbled something about having an unusual attack of nerves, hoping my honesty would make it go away. I asked someone else to take over and give the background on our meeting. A loyal employee, she looked worried but jumped in competently, adding to my crisis of self-confidence. I recovered somewhat after her preamble, but was distracted and sweaty, and my head was pounding through the rest of the meeting as I replayed the embarrassment over and over in my mind.

A senior employee dropped by to check on me later in the day, making it clear everyone had noticed and was concerned about my minor breakdown. "That was weird," he said, trying to reassure me that it was out of character. But his concern just reinforced my sense of inadequacy. I could not look anyone in the eye for several weeks as I envisioned that the shocking news of my visible meltdown had travelled to five hundred employees through the grapevine.

I had known that that particular job was taking its toll on my physical and emotional health, which is why I had left to take a job with a start-up competitor. Perhaps I had waited too long, and my cancer was a belated wake-up call.

Under siege

The year prior to my departure from Rogers had been spectacularly brutal. It started with a devastating round of staff layoffs. It was the third or fourth time I had been ordered to get up on the soap box to announce and defend organizational changes made by a new head office regime, as if I believed wholeheartedly in the new corporate direction. I was growing terribly weary of behaving as if I fully endorsed the decisions made by the current tenants in the corner suite. I felt like I was continually having to stand in front of jaded employees and "fake it" by promoting the flavour-of-the-month vision, spouting meaningless diatribe scripted by heartless, overpaid, cerebral executives who had spent no time in the trenches with these people. But I dutifully climbed onto the new bandwagon each time, feeling more and more like an impostor as I rallied the troops around the new ruling party's game plan. Instead of receiving the rulers' gratitude for championing the changes, I lived with the constant threat of losing my job if the new marching orders weren't well executed.

Perhaps symbolically, I lost my voice the day of the announcements, and could only croak out a painfully terse prepared statement.

In the middle of that year, my management team and I were asked to present our sales plans to a new team of young bucks from head office. They arrived with sharp pencils and, we soon realized, hidden agendas. I had not anticipated the cutthroat brutality of that session. We had been prepared for a collaborative dialogue between regional sales and head office marketing. But these accusators were single-mindedly determined to show up our incompetence rather than seek our input on the head office marketing programs. We walked out of the meeting completely humiliated.

Several weeks later, the president of a competitor called me to ask why his Sales VP had been approached by a headhunter for a job that sounded a lot like mine. My current boss had recently joined us from that competitor, and had a reputation for using others to promote his own interests. My guess was that he wanted to impress our current president by luring away the competitor's most senior sales executive – coincidentally also a close friend of his. Never mind if one of our people (me) became redundant in the process. His head office minions had just conveniently demonstrated my incompetence. My voice faltered as I tried to laugh the rumour off as a "fishing expedition", to save face with my competitor.

The next day, I got up the nerve to confront my boss about the headhunting foray. He stammered and avoided directly answering my question, which to me was all I needed to confirm that my job was in jeopardy. I stood up from my desk several days later and instantly felt a knife-like pain in my back – a muscle spasm – which left me semi-crippled for weeks. Apart from the obvious symbolism of being stabbed in the back, it is interesting that the pain was centred between my shoulder blades and radiated through to the centre of my chest – exactly where my cancer mass would be discovered a year and a half later.

Two further incidents added to my stress levels, just to finish me off. First, the company was caught up in a consumer outcry about a billing practice called "negative option", which allowed monthly charges to be renewed unless the customer took action to opt out. I had fought a lengthy internal battle to prevent the billing practice from being implemented. Ultimately, the decision had purportedly gone right up to Ted Rogers himself, and my objections had been overruled. Months later, as they saw the effects on their bills, our customers were predictably up in arms. It quickly escalated to become a media feeding frenzy. As the most senior western spokesperson, I was now expected to publicly defend the practice.

My office was under siege. Media headlines decried the company's unethical practices, accompanied by old file photos of me smiling – quite inappropriately, given the subject matter. I looked like a shifty corporate executive. This, combined with my puppet-like delivery of the approved media messages from head office, seemed to make me the local lightning rod for media and consumer indignation. I felt betrayed and crucified.

That was my pre-cancer world. I felt like I was surrounded by back-stabbing bosses, adversarial peers, frightened employees, bloodthirsty news media, irate customers and mutinous dealers. It became harder and harder to maintain my self-respect as I continued to abandon my own values in favour of keeping my job. I had all of the external trappings of power: big title, corner office, luxury car, expense account, hefty salary, bonuses and stock options – but I did not like the person I had become.

A welcome escape

I was delighted to be presented with the opportunity to leave it all behind and join a feisty little competitor with a much more values-based company culture. In fact, I felt quite vindicated in announcing my little coup before my boss was able to play out his plot to have me replaced. I spent the Friday before my resignation packing up my office and shredding files because I knew I'd be walked out of the building the minute I resigned. I called my boss's cell phone on a Sunday night hoping to leave a message to schedule a conversation the next morning. To my surprise, although it was close to midnight in Toronto, he answered his phone. When I requested the conversation, he insisted that we have it right then. After I blurted out my resignation, there was silence on the other end. And then, as expected, he quietly advised me not to bother coming in the next day. I confirmed that my keys and security pass were already on my desk along with my letter of resignation. It was all very courteous. After hanging up the phone, I danced a little jig, free of my oppressors once and for all.

I had the luxury of a few weeks off over Christmas before starting the new job. I enjoyed some rare family time, baking shortbread and making Christmas cakes with the kids, and focusing on meaningful gift-giving instead of the harried department store drive-by approach of prior years. Just after Christmas, I contracted a terrible virus and was finally forced to stop "doing" and just sleep for several days before starting the new job in January.

It was three months later, just as I was ramping up in the new role, that I found out I had cancer. I suddenly became the centre of well-meaning attention. I was showered with well wishes, prayers, compliments, love and encouragement. Even my former boss did me the honour of sending a very thoughtful message to my former colleagues, resulting in a flood of calls and letters from old friends. One of the most surprising was from Ted Rogers himself. He caught me off guard, on my cell phone, and after expressing his concern over my health, signed off with his characteristic "God bless".

I thought to myself how lucky I was to receive such an outpouring of compassion and positive energy. I wanted to always remember the healing effects of that energy, in contrast with the toxic impact of the blame, criticism, fear and animosity of my former job. Why could I not have recognized earlier that living in that state of constant anxiety was not a healthy place to be?

What I now see is that I seriously and almost irreversibly allowed my work to divert me from the person I wanted to be. As a child, I had been certain my life's calling was to serve others, to connect with people and make them better for having known me. Where had that gentle young girl gone? I was so busy playing the game, climbing the ladder, racing on the treadmill and living in fear that I had lost sight of what really mattered. I had thought work was my purpose. But, the work I had been doing (or, more accurately, the way I was doing it and perceiving it) was fundamentally on a disastrous collision course with my underlying values, my beliefs and my true purpose. The stresses of performing in an unforgiving corporate environment had reduced me to a self-protective, competitive and anxious workaholic.

As I completed my cancer-provoked self-analysis, I started to feel at peace with my situation. I knew, deep down, that the healing had started well before my diagnosis, when I had decided to change jobs. Now, I could use this illness as a door to stay in touch with my heart. Even while enduring the challenges of baldness, nausea, weight loss, early menopause, fatigue, chemo-brain, bone ache, and insomnia, I found I was able to approach my journey with a sense of adventure. I surrendered to the process, trying to savour every aspect of the experience to learn as much as I could.

Moving on with life

Nine months after diagnosis, I visited my oncologist and he declared me fully free of cancer. I felt that I had been given the gift of a second chance, and I vowed not to squander the lessons of my short-lived crisis.

To celebrate, Rob and I decided to go on a dream trip to London and Ireland. Rob had never really expressed his own fears during my treatment. His tacit strength had provided a welcome foundation for my courage. Now, clearly relieved to have his play-mate back, he had laboured for weeks to plan this holiday to the nth degree, booking beautiful Victorian castles and estates along our route. We stayed at five-star *Relais & Châteaux* from the *Michelin Guide* and indulged in decadent gourmet meals, creams and pastries as I tried to recoup some of my cancer weight loss. We enjoyed the fresh air of a riverboat on the Thames, operatic serenades at Covent Garden, and double decker bus tours of London. We drove the unnervingly narrow country roads of Ireland, and reveled in a horse and buggy ride through the mountains of Kerry.

Though weak, I felt very trendy with my bald pate and fancy hats. We took long walks in the mild British sunshine, and each day I grew stronger. During our last week we galloped on horseback across an emerald green field at Adare Manor in Ireland, and I felt truly free from disease and "emotional baggage". Life lay vibrantly ahead of us like the rolling green hills of the Irish countryside.

I went back to work full-time, went about the business of growing my hair back and moved on with my life. For the next few years, I enjoyed a highly successful career at Fido as we moved from start-up to earn an impressive share of the wireless market. I found a healthy balance between work and family time, and truly enjoyed my life. I worked with a team of folks who shared my values, in a company culture that was supportive and caring.

I had left my cancer well behind me, along with the stressful work environment I believed had made me susceptible to illness. But this was not the end of my healing journey – far from it.

4

BACK ON THE TREADMILL

Five years later, my life took another turn when I left my job with Fido. The company had been having financial difficulties and was centralizing its leadership team in Montreal. I had been offered the role of president, based in Montreal, but Rob and I were so committed to our Vancouver lifestyle that I turned it down. A new president was brought in, and over time the culture changed and started to resemble a context with which I was all too familiar. I watched the company evolve from a happy little start-up to just another large organization fraught with distrust and corporate politics.

For a while, I allowed myself to regress into the familiar pattern of overtime and frequent travel, driven by the fear of layoffs and job insecurity. I also instinctively reverted to the tough, competitive, self-protective persona I had honed in the Rogers environment, that person I did not like. I realized this type of corporate culture brought out the worst in me, and knew that I needed to escape before the pattern took its toll on my health. I negotiated a severance package as part of the downsizing. The company was disappointed that they couldn't find a role for me, but came up with a generous package for which I was grateful.

Hugely relieved, I ended my seventeen year career in the cell phone business. I set out onto the job market in 2002 with the intention of finding work that was a better fit for my soul. The severance package gave me the peace of mind to take some time to decide my next career move. I started by taking a few months off to get reacquainted with Rob and the kids. We took the holiday of a lifetime, starting with an idyllic week at Club Med on Lindeman Island on the Great Barrier Reef. We followed that with a one-week cruise up the coast of New Zealand. It was one of the true highlights of our lives. The kids were ten and twelve, just the right age to enjoy time with their parents. They also enjoyed the Club Med circus camps, and my heart soared when I watched them star in the high wire trapeze act in the "Big Show" on our final evening. All was right with the world at that moment.

When we returned home, I started my job search in a very tough market. I knew it would be a lengthy process to find something similar to my previous executive roles. It was 2002, and the massive downturn in the telecommunications and technology sectors had hit B.C. particularly hard. Eastern and U.S.-based companies had centralized their operations and downsized their branch offices, leaving Vancouver with a surplus of mid-career sales and marketing executives like me, all competing for scarce jobs.

My executive search

I investigated a variety of options. What do you do with an English degree, partial MBA and a decade and a half of experience promoting cell phones? As I talked to recruiters for advice, I recognized many were people like me, and I started to turn these interviews into research on a career in executive search. It looked like a decent fit for my interests and skills. There would be a steep learning curve and a strenuous investment in building a client base, but it had all the hallmarks of a good "second half" profession that would appeal to my desire to be in service to others. I loved the idea of helping great people find great jobs and helping great companies find great people.

After many interviews and a barrage of psychological profile tests, I was offered a position at Ray and Berndtson (now Boyden Executive Search), the largest executive search firm in Vancouver. It meant starting back at square one to learn a new trade and new skills. As daunting as that sounded, I had always been convinced I could excel at anything if I worked hard enough. Thus far, through my many roles and challenges, I had proven that to be true. I turned the same resolve and determination to the challenge of becoming a model student and high performer in my new career as a corporate recruiter.

In my typical hit-the-ground-in-overdrive fashion, I took on a volume of work and a pace I had not experienced since my early thirties. Being the obsessive, competitive overachiever that I am, I won the Rookie of the Year award in six months, and made partner in a year.

Being invited into the ranks of partner was a privilege. Along with the prestige came the expectation that I would produce at an even higher volume level. Perhaps the most unforgiving expectation was my own. Each week when the new business numbers were published at the partners' meetings, I would beat myself up for not being in the top three. Never mind that the other partners had been building their practices for as long as five, ten, twenty or even thirty years. I was not that patient with myself. Since every other challenge I had taken on had been conquered through sheer hard work, I just ramped up my pace, putting in twelve-hour days at the office, taking work home every evening and weekend, and hauling two full briefcases on my frequent business trips.

Somehow, it seemed to me that the more tenured partners made a similar number of assignments look easier. I came to realize that was because they had earned the right to delegate a significant amount of the work to the more junior consultants. As a rookie, I was a "delegatee" rather than a "delegator". I was grateful to support the senior partners on their accounts, in order to learn the business and earn income while building my own roster. I invested a lot of time and energy into growing my own clients, while willingly carrying the load on as many of the partners' searches as I was invited to take on.

An Olympian challenge

My business development efforts finally started to bear fruit at a time when I was supporting a peak number of searches for my partners. My workload virtually doubled in the span of a few months. But that was not all; just when I thought I could not possibly take on more work, I was invited to work with our managing partner, Kyle Mitchell, on the most prestigious and politically sensitive new business pitch the firm had made in years: recruiting the CEO and senior leadership team for the Vancouver Organizing Committee for the Olympics. We invested hours in brainstorming, analyzing and documenting our approach, followed by rehearsals and rethinks to craft our presentation. We won the pitch against stiff competition, resulting in seven immediate new assignments. After the initial exhilaration of the win, I felt like a deer in the headlights, frozen with panic at how I was going to shoehorn this politically-sensitive and highly demanding work into my already chaotic schedule.

As with most challenges I had faced, I knew the answer was simply to work harder. I started my days with 6 a.m. conference calls to interview eastern candidates; I devoted my evenings to business development events or client entertainment. I worked at least one day each weekend, compressing my quality family time into Sundays when I wasn't travelling. I squeezed my exercise routine into this bloated agenda by running the four miles to and from the office with a backpack full of work clothes.

Just to add to this, when I was hired I had agreed to take on the role of Administrative Partner, as part of a succession plan to Managing Partner. This involved organizing partners' meetings, mentoring the administrative and marketing staff, and planning business development strategies for the firm.

Somehow, through sheer determination and hard work, I finally built my revenues enough to rank in the top three for at least one quarter. It was briefly satisfying, but my relentless quest for success was taking its toll on my family life and my mental state. What was it about me that I needed to turn every work experience into a competitive race to the finish?

Out of balance

It was around this time that I discovered an entry Maddie made in her diary. I had found it under the comforter when making her bed. I would not normally even think of reading her personal diary, but it fell open to the most recent page, where in her artistic, confident printing she had written, "I have to spend time with my mom this week because she's gonna take some days off work. I like spending time with her because I never get to. She's always at work!"

It made my heart hurt. Maddie was already twelve, and Conor was fourteen. They would not be interested in spending time with me for very much longer, and here I was blowing my brains out at a job rather than investing a fraction of that energy into something vastly more important to me. I had lapsed back into the familiar pattern of work-dominated overdrive that I had vowed to avoid after my first cancer scare. Was I in danger of squandering that precious reminder about what was really important? I promised myself to find a way to get back to a healthier balance.

Six months later, however, I was relieved of the responsibility of making good on that promise. Through an absurd set of circumstances, I was plunged into a surreal life-and-death drama that completely changed the ground rules.

5

THE CASE OF THE MISSING TOENAILS

Scene One

We see the walk-in closet of our Heroine and Husband. The couple are preparing for a black tie event for which they are apparently running late.

Heroine enters, barefoot and panicky, in a semi-clad flap, clenching a toothbrush in one hand, wearing hair curlers, and applying an eyelash curler with the other hand.

She speaks incessantly and obsessively, partially addressing the Husband who is wife-deaf in some other room, but mostly nattering to herself while fishing around in the closet.

"Once again, I have no shoes to wear.

"Another frigging, obligatory black tie affair, and it's bad enough that I have to drag out one of you old, tired, dusty evening gowns skulking in the back of the closet like spinsters awaiting an infrequent suitor. Which of you will be kind to the tummy pouch and hips this year? Never mind, it is the shoes that really matter, and I am simply screwed in that department.

"There you are, my proud, madcap-splurge, last-season designer shoes, twinkling up at me, ever hopeful. You are my glass slippers-in-waiting, ready to transform the charwoman to the princess and carry me out to a night of inspired magic. Oh how I yearn for the barefoot freedom of my beautifully bejeweled and nearly naked Stuart Weitzman sandals.

"But it is not to be. It is not simply that I need a pedicure; it is that at this precise moment I actually have NO big toenails. Just wizened calluses with remnants of some dark polish that makes them look like the raisins you find in the furnace vents. This week just whizzed by, and I didn't give any thought to the state of my feet. I certainly had no time to rush down to the pedicurist to get a pair of what I call my 'podiatric prostheses'.

"Why have I been caught nail-less, you might ask? Because, for the past seven years since I had chemotherapy, my big toenails have fallen off, frustratingly, every spring – just in time for open-toed shoe season. My solution has been to rush down to the nail bar and get acrylic toenails. Equally frustratingly, these do not usually last for more than two or three naked toe outings. This year, both acrylic toenails gleefully abandoned me on my first joyful early spring romp on the beach. They quietly burrowed themselves into the sand as I trudged on, oblivious to their departure until much later when I went to rinse the sand off, only to discover the appalling defection.

"Hopefully, the AWOL offenders were not later mistaken for seashells by a foraging seagull and rejected mid-air, only to land in all of their crimson-lacquered glory in some poor child's French fries!"

The Heroine turns her attention back to the closet and the practical matter of finding footwear.

"I am sick and tired of making do with pumps or sling-backs when everyone else is showing off perfect prosthetic-free pedicures every summer! It is also not fair that I can't claim my artificial appendages on my extended health care plan. In my view, they are legitimate medical expenses – after all, it was medical treatment that caused the problem in the first place! My hair is back to normal, my weight is back to normal, even the stupid stubble on my legs came back in thickets – but *no toenails.* As far as I am concerned, that legitimately qualifies as Accidental Dismemberment!

"Oh well, I guess I can't really complain if that is the only lingering effect of my cancer treatment. Who am I to get my vanity in a knot about the state of my pedicure? I should be thankful to be here at all!

"(Note to self: make appointment with GP to get a prescription for antifungal medicine that will solve the problem once and for all. Vanity prevails!)"

Throughout this monologue, Heroine has managed to select and don a gown, remove hair curlers, apply deodorant, mascara and lipstick, and is now brandishing a pair of decidedly matronly sling-back shoes.

Tuxedoed and obviously irritable Husband enters, looking beyond impatient.

"Are you ready yet? We are now half an hour late," he growls.

"Just look at these shoes!" our heroine bemoans.

"Lovely, sweetheart. Let's go."

Scene Two

It is several weeks later. We see the examining room of a typical doctor's office. Heroine is re-buttoning her blouse, sitting on the examining table while the physician madly scribbles notes before looking her directly in the eye over his spectacles.

Doctor: "I'm afraid I don't have very good news for you, my dear. As you know we did the blood test to see if you can take the antifungal medicine to treat your toenails. We called you back in to discuss the results of that blood test, which are not good. Your enzyme levels are elevated, and from the examination it appears that your spleen is enlarged. I will have to send you for more tests, and I am referring you to a gastroenterologist."

Heroine, obviously not grasping the gravity of the situation: "What do I do about my toenails?"

Doctor: "I should think that would be the least of your concerns right now."

Heroine: "But, what are you telling me?"

Doctor: "Well, I am not a liver specialist, but these readings could indicate some form of hepatitis, bile duct blockage, or they could be an anomaly. Since you tell me you are not a heavy drinker (eyebrow raised), it is probably not alcohol-related cirrhosis (other eyebrow raised), though the readings are similar and you do appear to be a bit jaundiced."

Heroine, to audience: – "How much is heavy … those two – okay three – glasses of wine twice a week? Or are we worried about those Tequila parties back in high school? And I certainly haven't noticed any jaundice – but then, I do have a pretty good tan this year."

Doctor: "Is there any history of liver disease in your family?

"No."

"Have you been tested for Hepatitis?"

"No."

"Any history of Wilson's disease or Hemachromatosis or other genetic disorders?"

"No!" (*Heroine appears at this stage to be nobly repressing imminent hysteria.*)

"I will send the referral to the specialist today, and I expect his office will call you next week. I want you to take this requisition to the lab immediately for blood and urine tests, so that he has something to go by. I am sorry about this, I know you did not come here because you felt ill, but after not seeing the medical community for some time, it looks like you might be seeing a bit more of us for a while."

Heroine, to audience: "Why is this man smiling?"

Scene Three

Several weeks later. We are in another typical doctor's office. Receptionist is answering telephone. Large clock on wall says 9:49.

Heroine rushes in, breathless, ending cell call. "Okay, start the meeting without me if I'm running late." Heroine then addresses medical assistant: "Hi, it's me, my appointment is for 9:30, sorry I'm late."

Receptionist: "That's fine. Please take a seat."

Heroine: "Do you know if the doctor has received my lab results? The ultrasound was done last Saturday."

Receptionist: "I don't think so. I'll check with the lab to see if they're available."

Heroine [to audience]: "I know they're available because I already phoned the lab and they said they had sent them to the doctor's office. Dare I say this and further alienate the gatekeeper? Perhaps not."

Time passes, clock ticks loudly. At 10:05 a.m. the receptionist invites another patient in.

Heroine, visibly annoyed, addresses receptionist: "I do have another appointment back downtown at 10:30 – do you think I should be canceling it, or should I come back another time?"

Receptionist: "Well, you were late."

Heroine: "Yes, but that was half an hour ago. Does the doctor know I'm here?"

Receptionist: "He's with another patient."

Heroine: "Was their appointment before mine?"

Receptionist: "No, but they were here first".

Heroine: "I'll postpone my 10:30 appointment then."

Receptionist: "That's up to you."

Time passes. The clock now says 10:22 a.m.

Receptionist: "The doctor will see you now."

Heroine: "Do you know if he has my lab results now?"

Receptionist: "I'll check with the lab."

Scene Four

Inside another typical examining room. Heroine is sitting on the examining table, re-buttoning her blouse.

Gastroenterologist: "Well, your liver is in some trouble, the spleen seems enlarged, you appear slightly jaundiced, but without your lab results, it's hard to tell what's going on."

Heroine, sweetly, between clenched teeth: "I would think the lab results may be here by now; your receptionist has had an hour to track them down."

Just then, efficient receptionist rushes in with a fax report and plunks it down in front of the doctor. His brow furrows, he looks first alarmed, then surprised. Then his face softens into a kind, compassionate mask as he frames his next words:

"My dear, given what I see on this ultrasound report, I believe I would like to refer you back to your oncologist."

Heroine, to audience: "He's got to be kidding! From absent toenails to cancer relapse? I don't even feel sick."

6

WE HAVE REACHED OUR
TERMINAL DESTINATION

And so starts Round Two. My cancer reprieve had lasted a full seven years. Here I am, facing the news that I am sick again – so sick that my liver is seriously compromised. My gastroenterologist suspects that I have a recurrence of cancer that has progressed to the liver, and refers me directly to my oncologist rather than prescribing additional liver tests.

I am incredulous. I wonder how I could possibly be as ill as my doctors think I am, and not have noticed any symptoms. I refuse to believe that my cancer has returned. I fully expect the doctors to find that I have some virus or maybe a mild form of hepatitis that can be easily treated.

The diagnostic rollercoaster

On my first visit to my oncologist, he examines me and orders the usual tests, but he seems to agree with my theory that it is not cancer that is causing the liver distress, and promptly sends me back to the gastroenterologist to investigate further.

But my original gastroenterologist is on vacation, so I become the problem of another specialist. Like the first one, this man also strongly suspects that it is cancer that is causing the liver problems, given my history. He wants me to go back and see the oncologist. I am starting to get frustrated at this game of medical ping pong. I really don't care which of these physicians sorts out the problem, as long as someone does. I had naively assumed that all medical practitioners were interested in the whole process from diagnosis through treatment and prevention. It feels, instead, like neither of these specialists wants to assume responsibility for my care until there is a confirmed diagnosis. I am quickly learning that I will have to be the one to take some initiative if any progress is to be made. I push both specialists to order whatever tests are necessary to diagnose the source of my liver distress.

As the results of each test come through, I visit first the gastro-enterologist and then the oncologist to try to gain some insight on what they are finding. But each visit just seems to lead to more questions and more tests, in a process that appears to have no end in sight. The most difficult part of this diagnostic rollercoaster lies in getting information on what is really going on. I envision my paperwork accumulating in overburdened in-baskets, like chapters in a manuscript, which could reveal the whole story if only someone took the time to read them.

After several months of incessant and inconclusive tests, I am starting to look and feel more and more ill. My belly is now distended and I am quite jaundiced. Finally my gastroenterologist refers me to a surgeon for a laparoscopic biopsy of the liver.

Double jeopardy

Days later, I listen with increasing incredulity as my GP explains that I have a relapse of Hodgkin's Disease which has progressed beyond the chest area to several lymph nodes adjacent to my liver. "*What?*" Until this moment, I had never really allowed myself to believe that my cancer could be back.

"And I expect you know," my GP continues, "that your liver biopsy revealed Stage 4 cirrhosis – irreversible liver damage. I am not sure if they've told you what treatment you will require, but in my experience it eventually means a transplant."

Then, with a puzzled look, he further explained that the liver disease and the cancer appeared to be unrelated. "It seems you are one very unlucky lady," he summarizes.

I felt like I have been punched in my swollen gut. No, *seriously*, I wonder, how plausible could it be that I have *two* "unrelated", potentially fatal medical conditions fighting for supremacy in my poor bloated body? I am not sure whether to cry or laugh at the total absurdity of this situation.

I call Rob and somehow convey the situation to him over the phone in a fairly calm manner. Poor Rob; it is the second time in our twenty year marriage that he has received the news that I have a life-threatening diagnosis. His reaction now is the same as before, and so many times since. Strong, cheerful, encouraging and sympathetic, all in one loving tone of voice. "We'll get through this." Thank God for him.

Stepping off the treadmill

Rob's reassurance gives me the strength to call the office. I have decided, in an instant, that I am going to take a leave of absence. Though I worked right through my treatments with my first cancer diagnosis, this time I realize I will have to give my full attention to my health. This time the cancer has apparently progressed much further, and of course there is the inexplicable condition of my liver. Even though I expect to heal quickly from the biopsy symptoms and soon be well enough to work, I tell myself it would be insane to try to continue as if nothing is wrong.

Caroline, my kind mentor at the firm, is audibly shaken by my news. I realize in that moment how truly serious the situation is. This is not just "calling in sick" with the potential of returning in a few weeks' time. There is the serious potential that I will not be returning, period. I think until I had spoken the words "my cancer is back" out loud to a real person, I had felt like this was happening to someone else, like I was watching a TV show and would be able to turn it off when it was over. I had no inkling of the extent to which the concept of "normal life" could be altered for me forever.

Caroline wisely counsels me not to make any rash decisions while in the hospital, such as taking an extended leave of absence. "There's lots of time for that," she says. "Right now you should just rest and not worry about this place for a while. Let's just see how things go."

But I cannot ignore an overwhelming sense of relief that I may not have to go back to work, at least for a while. My unexpected diagnosis feels like an involuntary hall pass, a fate-imposed permission slip to get off the treadmill. Why was it that once again, I had to wait for such a drastic situation to give myself that permission?

After my release from the hospital, I immediately make an appointment to see my oncologist, determined to have my GP's version of the facts validated by at least one of my specialists.

"I am not sure," he begins. "It is possible this cancer is dormant, possibly remaining from your first occurrence." This seems like more of a question than an answer. But, he explains, it is concerning that they have found cancer cells in the lymph nodes adjacent to the liver, as this means it has progressed to Stage III, well beyond the Stage II diagnosis of my first bout with Hodgkins. "Perhaps we missed something," he wonders. He seems to be talking more to himself than to me, trying to decipher the clues. Perhaps, he continues, these cells were present all along – in which case if it was active, it was a very slow form of cancer. Like me, the kind doctor seems to be unwilling to entertain the possibility that I have recurrent, active lymphoma. With his next statement, though, I realize this may be partly hope on his part rather than science. "In any event, we cannot treat the cancer as it would destroy what is left of your liver. You need to see your gastroenterologist so he can diagnose and treat the liver problem. We will hope that he can find a way to improve the condition of the liver, so that if the cancer is not dormant, the liver can tolerate some form of chemotherapy."

Despite the ambiguity of this diagnosis, I like the oncologist's approach. I like the fact that he leaves doors of hope open as he walks through the situation with us. It is easier to hear "your cancer might be dormant" and "we will hope the liver can be improved" than the possible reality that my cancer cannot be treated.

Clinging to these kernels of optimism, I make an appointment to see the gastroenterologist. The doctor who has been treating me since the toenail incident is still on vacation, so I call the GI who visited me in the hospital. The one time slot he has available that week coincides with an important client meeting for Rob, and I desperately want company for this important consultation with yet another unfamiliar specialist. I ask my sister Carol to join me. It's not like she doesn't also have a busy schedule as she is a provincial court judge, but the appointment happily falls on her day off. I fill her in on the situation, and we arrive at the doctor's office buoyed by the hope instilled by my oncologist. We soon discover, however, that this new doctor's approach is not nearly as positive. In the absence of a definitive diagnosis, he does not fill in the blanks with hopeful possibilities. The few words he chooses to utter are not words of encouragement.

No way out?

I am immensely grateful to have my sister Carol's company to be my "back-up brain". We are identical twins, very similar in our approach, but her legal training gives her a more forensic perspective that I greatly admire. She is able to formulate the straight questions. She is also more confident around authority than me, and is therefore able to ask those straight questions with an assumption of stature that commands a straight answer. I'm not sure if it is the doctor's recognition of her status as a fellow professional, or just that he is responding to her practiced judiciary tone, but this taciturn doctor suddenly finds his voice when she looks him in the eye and starts her line of questioning. While I resent the inference that he thinks she is the more important twin, it has the desired effect.

We are hoping to glean some clues about what is causing the liver condition and how it can be treated. However, the doctor advises us that despite all of the testing, it is not possible to pinpoint the cause of my liver disease. It is not that unusual, he says, for people to be diagnosed with liver disorders after several decades of undetected illness. The cause could be a long-ago virus which triggered an autoimmune response; or prolonged exposure to toxins; or a genetically inherited disease. When the exact cause cannot be identified and cannot be labeled as Hepatitis A, B or C, it is referred to as "cryptogenic" or "idiopathic" – of unknown origin.

Even if it cannot be identified, he continues, most liver disorders can be treated with steroids to stop the disease from progressing. Some people can live for "a number of years" on a compromised liver, he adds. This appears to be the equivalent of wild optimism from this undemonstrative professional. Even though the liver will *never recover*, he continues, the various symptoms of cirrhosis can be managed, and under normal circumstances, some people are able to maintain a good quality of life for 5 to 10 years or possibly more. At this point I am finding his generalized references to "some people" and "normal circumstances" to be highly annoying. *Why isn't he talking about me?* I wonder. I soon find out.

"However", he states, as if it is a sentence. "In your case, it is clear that the liver is rapidly deteriorating, probably because of the interaction with your Hodgkin's disease. If this continues you will soon need a liver transplant." He utters the words in a clinical tone that makes the inconceivable sound routine.

"However," he says. *Another* however? That can't be good, I realize. At this point the doctor pauses, as if to punctuate the finality of his next remark. "You are not eligible for a liver transplant because you have active cancer. I'm sorry."

I interpret the words "I'm sorry" to mean he believes he has finished the story. But I am having trouble understanding what he is saying. He has not explained why I am not eligible for what is apparently the only treatment that can save my life. Then Carol and I both come to the same conclusion at the same time: this man is implying that the medical system views me as "not worth the risk" because I have another life-threatening condition. In their view I am already potentially terminal from my cancer, so I am not a good bet for a rare and expensive life-saving procedure for another condition. In this man's medically trained view, I am destined to be an unfortunate casualty in a world of triage where scarce resources are not wasted on high risk patients.

Carol decides to cross-examine for more information: "What is the alternative?"

"I don't know," he replies. "I think we should do more tests to see if we can do a better job of pinpointing the cause of the hepatitis, so we can determine if there is any treatment to slow its progress." He does not sound very hopeful.

7

A Comedy of Errors

So there it was. I had gone from the double whammy of having two life-threatening diseases, to the triple threat of knowing each made the other untreatable. I no longer felt relieved about having an involuntary hall-pass to take time off work. Instead, I felt scared that I may have found myself an exit strategy with no way back to the main highway after the rest stop.

On the way home, Carol tried to bolster me with cheerful encouragement, invoking the constitutional family belief that things will always work out.

Back home, alone for once, I put on the kettle and tried to busy myself with normal household routines but my thoughts were caught up in how I would tell Rob, Conor and Maddie that things were not looking very good. All I could see around me was the lifeless house: breakfast dishes stacked in the sink; the unoccupied, unmade bed – normal things to remind me that nothing at all was normal.

I was forty-seven. Maddie was in Grade 7, Conor in Grade 9. Where had the time gone? I could not remember the names of their teachers. I didn't know if they would be coming home right after school, or visiting with friends. Did Maddie have a soccer practice? Was Conor going to his volunteer work?

I suddenly realized that I had been so totally preoccupied with the demands of my medical reality that it had become my new full-time occupation. In fact, it was a 24/7 preoccupation, and it dawned on me that my family had learned to function without my full involvement, as if my illness was just another job. Despite being off work, I had been so caught up in my diagnostic ordeal for the past five months that I had absented myself from my own life, in the interest of trying to save it. Worse, I had no idea how my sweet children and supportive husband might be feeling about the situation.

Between my silent worrying and my desperate drive to act normal to avoid alarming my family, I had unwittingly distanced myself from the one source of solace I needed most in this time of darkness. The kettle screamed on the stove as I sank my head into my hands and wept.

By the time everyone had come home I was slightly more composed. Maddie bounced in to ask for help with her homework. I cheerfully and willingly pitched in, while Conor and Rob sat with us in the family room watching *The Simpsons*. Fully present for once, I savoured the moment of domestic ordinariness, and held back the tears.

The next day I was full of resolve. It was not in me to give up, even when my medical team was not offering a lot of hope. I decided to remain so positive in my interactions with my doctors that they would have no choice but to believe my conviction that a solution would be found. I knew there was a difficult road ahead, with more tests and uncertainty, and I decided to embrace that reality. I welcomed each new procedure as it would take me closer to solving the mystery. Each was an opportunity to understand more about how to navigate the complexity of the medical system, and I often learned a lot about what questions I should have asked in advance.

This won't hurt a bit

One example was my first gastroscopy, which was used to diagnose the progress of my liver disease. The doctor administering the operation assured me that the procedure would be short and efficient, and the recovery time would be minimal because it only required a local anesthetic. After everything else I had been through it sounded like a piece of cake.

But apparently I did not ask all the right questions about what was involved. I had focused on his reassuring words such as "routine", "short", "efficient", "simple and painless". I forgot to ask about other words like nasty, nauseating, humiliating and ghastly. I had leapt to the assumption that this scope would be simple. After all, it didn't even have its own acronym, unlike other procedures I had encountered such as the ERCP, MRI, ECG or CT. My theory was that the clever medical professionals who dream up all of this jargon believe that short unintelligible acronyms make really unpleasant procedures sound less threatening to us unsuspecting patients.

So I assumed that since "gastroscopy" didn't rate its own four letter word, it couldn't be that bad. In retrospect, I am now certain it must have one; they just didn't tell me what it was. In fact, I know deep in my heart, stomach and esophagus that it must have a really unpleasant four letter, onomatopoeic acronym. Something like: Gastro-Analytic-Guessing-Game (GAGG); or Preliminary Unanaesthetized Kinetic Examination (PUKE). Or worse, perhaps it had an even longer epithet: "Unpleasant Procedure Causing Humiliation, Urination, Coughing & Kicking (UPCHUCK).

As usual, I arrive armed with a good book.

After a kind nurse brings me a warm blanket, I am lulled into a false sense of security, and I actually settle into a pleasant nap. No one tells me why I am waiting or how long it might be, or what horrors lie ahead.

After a very long wait, the OR nurse comes in and advises me that they have finally located the doctor, who has finally located his briefcase. I didn't know that either had been missing.

Finally, we begin. The OR Nurse gives me a small cup filled with a vile red liquid. She insists that I gargle until I gag and then swallow the whole mess. Quickly I cannot feel my throat and my esophagus. When could I ever feel my esophagus? I wonder – but all that is about to change.

The doctor asks me to suck on a small breathing ring, sort of like a hard plastic soother. He then whips out a clear plastic tube that looks like a dishwasher hose. It is inserted through the breathing ring and makes a probing assault on my anaesthetized throat.

It quickly becomes apparent that local anesthesia does not prevent the gag reflex. It may, in fact, exacerbate it. This does not seem to surprise or disturb the doctor or the nurse, who actually compliment me on how well I am doing, as I gag my way through the act of swallowing several inches of hose.

Back in the recovery room, feeling violated, I am visited by an old family friend who happens to be a nurse and just happens to be on shift in this ward. I shall call her "Joy" as that is what seems to characterize her cheery presence in the room – and because that is also her name. Joy exudes reassurance, wisdom and experience. When she discovers I had not opted for the alternative to local anesthesia – "conscious sedation" (a pleasant short departure into dreamland), she remarks on how brave I am.

What she does not know until I set her straight, is that no one had actually offered me the choice between being brave or taking the meds. Apparently she is quite familiar with the effects of the less-recommended, unmedicated approach, because her next comment is "I expect you'll be needing some fresh panties then," and off she bustles to find a handy disposable pair.

I gratefully accept the proffered garment, and try to regain enough dignity and composure to venture back into the changing room with the paper panties rustling beneath my hospital gown.

Note to self: ask about sedation for future procedures.

A glimmer of hepatic hope

Shortly after this vile procedure, the doctor who had administered the probe redeemed himself in my eyes forever. After completing my gastroscopic assault, he apparently spent the balance of the day reading my file and searching the Internet for a correlation between liver disease and Hodgkin's lymphoma. He was able to come up with a theory that warranted further investigation. Not only did he undertake to do this on his own time, he called me at home that evening to excitedly describe his findings and to refer me to a leading hepatologist, to whom he had already sent my file. This, in my jaded view of the system, was close to a miracle. This wonderfully caring and optimistic man was not even my primary gastroenterologist at the time. I quickly rectified that. It was probably one of the best moves I made in the whole course of my treatment.

We scheduled the earliest possible appointment with the hepatologist. Inevitably, it was nearly a month away.

Exhausted after all of the diagnostic ordeals, we took a two-week family summer vacation to Savary Island. A co-worker of Rob's and a good friend kindly offered us the opportunity to rent their fabulous waterfront cottage. It was a poignant, bittersweet holiday. Despite being physically frail, I had enough strength to participate in our outings, and enjoyed every moment of time with the kids and Rob. We drank the fresh air, swam in the warm ocean, jumped off the dock, walked and biked up and down the island, dug for clams and made homemade clam chowder. We had many happy nights at the island restaurant, biking all the way down the hill to our beach house in the pitch dark with only our flashlights and occasional moonlight to guide us.

If it weren't for the spectre of my illness, it would have been the happiest time of our lives.

8

THE ASSERTIVE PATIENT

I returned from our poignant vacation hell-bent on fighting for my life. I was entering month five of the diagnostic journey with no clear game plan, and I was afraid that my two diseases were making faster progress than my medical team.

I quickly realized that if I didn't take charge of this mess, no one would. While each of my specialists was working to solve their piece of the puzzle, they were working in silos. They were in two different health authorities whose systems did not talk to each other. Neither was the ultimate project leader, and we still had not reached the point where anyone had offered any hope for treatment. I had spent much of my career driving project teams to meet accelerated delivery schedules, and I was worried at the lack of coordination and efficiency on this job, where the stakes were literally life or death – mine! It was time to take control. My corporate instincts had gone into high alert.

Throughout my personal and professional life, I had always believed that having a positive plan was 90% of the battle. After my promotion to VP at the age of thirty-two, I had been invited to give a speech on my career success. The title was "Life is a Self-fulfilling Prophesy". I told the story of how each of my written five-year plans had somewhat miraculously come to be, almost to the letter.

Yet since the beginning of this health journey, I had not taken my own advice. Why was I allowing my fear to sideline my conviction that I could manifest a similar positive, self-fulfilling outcome for my healing? And so, finally, I sat down to write the plan. What emerged was in some ways absurd, but it was a cathartic use of my business skills and an outlet for my drive to conquer this ultimate challenge.

A preposterous plan

Project: Heal Kathy McLaughlin

Goal: Achieve complete cancer remission with minimal side effects, and restore liver to full functionality by end of fiscal year.

Action Plan:

1. Assemble team: ensure the right people on the bus: find a gastroenterologist for a second opinion

2. Ensure the team knows the key goals and KPIs
    Responsibility: KMc – End of month

3. Provide positive encouragement for team and individuals' progress – KMc, ongoing

4. Complete diagnostic phase by end of First Quarter/05
    Responsibility: oncologist, gastroenterologist

5. Decide on course of treatment
    Responsibility: GI – liver; Onc – Cancer; KMc veto or second opinion

6. Treat liver to stop progression of autoimmune disorder by end of Second Quarter/05 and fortify liver to withstand chemo
    Responsibility: GI

7. Determine cancer treatment plan and schedule (concurrent – by end of Second Quarter /05)
   Responsibility: Onc

8. Execute cancer treatment plan to achieve a minimum 80% reduction in malignant mass by end of fourth quarter; full remission by end of First Quarter /06
   Responsibility: Onc

9. Leave liver, lungs, etc. in functional condition; no further treatment required.
   Responsibility: Onc, KMc, GP, respirologist, etc.

Of course, the problem with having a project plan like this is that you need willing team members to participate. Insisting to an oncologist that he should cure you by First Quarter/06 would have been like asking the Queen to bring you tea at 2 p.m. Not only presumptuous, but preposterous. So my impudent directive sat in my journal. But the sheer act of writing it had given me a renewed sense of purpose, a conviction that I would do all I could to provide leadership and motivate my so-called team to achieve a happy outcome.

Absurd as it was, I believe that having that plan saved me – at least psychologically – from the fate of many I witnessed around me, who innocently entrusted their care to a chaotic and overburdened system. As I observed my fellow patients, I developed a huge amount of compassion for those who did not have the training, experience or determination to do the same for themselves. I saw many bewildered, naïve or surrendered patients who had given up their power to others. They seemed frustrated, yet continued to put their trust in "the system," assuming they were powerless to insist on better care. But to me, fighting for my life was not the time to be submissive.

I am lucky: I arrived in life blessed with a healthy dose of assertiveness combined with what my friends have referred to as pathological optimism. (My sister has been known to refer to it as obscene optimism.) This assertive optimism had always served me well whenever I was the one who had control of my choices. In this situation, however, it would have been easy to accept the reality that my fate was in other hands. I realized that the daunting task at hand was to cheerfully convince my medical experts that there was hope for a solution at the end of this journey, in the face of very poor medical odds.

No retreat, no surrender

The medical community is growing more accustomed to assertive patients, but we are still not the norm.

In the medical world, "care" is quite different from "service". Care requires a surrendered patient. For those of us who are assertive customers, it is hard to be cared for. Even for those who like being surrendered patients (and there seems to be a number of those in the system), it is a fine line between patient and victim in a system that doesn't have a lot of time for care.

It is also tough to be an assertive customer with medical professionals who are trained to be knowledgeable experts. Experts do not like to have their knowledge questioned. Doctors are trained to "know more" than their patients. Informed patients are sometimes threatening. Yet, with the wealth of medical information available electronically, it is relatively easy to become knowledgeable about one's specific medical diagnosis. It is even possible to acquire deeper and more up-to-date information on current treatments and outcomes than some of the specialists, who are overwhelmingly busy and are required to be knowledgeable across a broad spectrum within their field.

All of this leads to a rather interesting set of possibilities, especially when you run into a physician who has not encountered your situation before. If you are not used to asking the tough questions (Have you treated this set of symptoms with any success in the past?

What is the expected success rate of this treatment? What are the other options?) you may receive a decision that sounds like it is the only answer available for your situation. And if you do ask the tough questions, you may alienate your expert-doctors to the point that they don't feel like being all that helpful. You don't want to do that.

I remember reading somewhere that patients whose doctors "like" them have a higher chance of recovery. To me, that just makes sense: your doctor has to be on your team, standing for your success, in order to try their hardest to win. So, I realized that I needed to find the appropriate balance of assertion and friendly respect to win over each of my medical practitioners. For me, this was especially difficult if they did not have a sense of humour. Thankfully, most did.

Ultimately, what I learned about survival in the "system" was that every patient has rights, but it is up to the patient to enforce them. You have the right to ask a lot of questions. You have the right to ask for a second opinion and even a third. You have the right to say no to some procedures and treatments. And, most of all, you have the right to remain positive and expect positive outcomes.

Copy that

Another lesson I learned on my journey as an assertive patient navigating through the labyrinth of testing was to request copies of my medical reports. At first, my request was often denied. It was unusual at that time for patients to receive copies of their reports, and it was well before the enlightened era when one could obtain online access to test results. None of the labs or technicians was able to release copies of information to me; it was up to the ordering physician to do so. I learned that I could ask the doctor to write "copy to patient" on the requisition for the more routine tests, and eventually I might receive a copy in the mail. For the more sensitive or complex doctors' reports, I had to request a photocopy from the doctor's medical office assistant. Many were not comfortable doing this for fear the patient would misinterpret the information. I had to reassure them that it was not for self-diagnosis, but for record keeping as I had so many specialists who asked questions about my procedures.

In the case of tests done at my local hospital, I found out there was a personal information release form I could sign requesting my patient records for a specific period of time; I got in the habit of doing this once every few months, and received a one and a half inch file of paper in the mail six weeks later. This gave me the added benefit of receiving post-procedure reports with the detailed results of various scopes, CT scans, MRIs and other tests, including the reviewing expert's written analysis of the results.

Patients rarely see these documents, probably for good reason as they are written in "medlish", a secret language only decipherable by physicians who have studied for years to learn the medical vernacular. While I was able to use the Internet to decode most of the cryptic narrative, the information arrived long after it would have been most helpful in tracking the progress of my treatment. I can only hope that future generations of patient navigators will have freer access to their data.

I realize that not everyone wants to keep this level of detail on their health test results, but I am not one to close my eyes and hope for the best. I needed to be proactive, to take control of what I thought I could influence, and ensure nothing fell through the cracks.

I found it immensely reassuring each time I had to see a new specialist, to be able to hand over my neatly organized, chronological binder and know that they had the full audit trail of my situation. Usually they were pleasantly surprised and quite grateful. Prior to figuring this out, I had been appalled to learn that many of my specialists seemed to have very limited information on me when I arrived as a new patient. This was partly because I was being treated in two health regions. For some bureaucratic reason, they did not provide each other with access to each other's patient records at that time. This was both frustrating and frightening. Frustrating because it was time-consuming for me to always have to fill in the story in response to a barrage of questions. Frightening, because it could actually be life-threatening if some significant detail was overlooked.

Armed with my take-charge healing plan and meticulously organized binder, I started proactively calling my doctors to inquire about the outcomes of various tests. I cheerily encouraged their assistants to squeeze me into their appointment books rather than wait several weeks between tests. During visits, I continued to positively insist that things were going well, we were going to get to the bottom of this, I was certain we could figure it out. Even when the doctors looked puzzled or concerned, I gently cajoled them into good humour and tried to influence them with my optimism.

A lot of questions, and some answers

Finally, the time came to see the hepatologist. Rob and I went to the appointment together.

The hepatologist was the first specialist to give us a glimmer of hope. He had deduced that I had an autoimmune liver disorder probably caused by a tropical disease contracted fifteen or twenty years ago. The undetected disease had been slowly progressing since before my first bout of lymphoma. The liver had tolerated the chemo treatments, but had sustained further damage, still undetected.

Now, the second onset of Hodgkin's had exacerbated the liver distress to the point of serious compromise. If his theory was right, he believed that the liver could be treated with steroids to get back to its "pre-relapse" level of dysfunction, well enough to tolerate another course of chemotherapy. In the overall scheme of things, we thought this was pretty good news. I think even the doctor cracked a smile.

Trial and error

I was started on a dose of 80 mg of Prednisone daily. I was to stay on this potent steroid until mid-December, when, if the liver was responding adequately, I could start chemotherapy. Finally, we were getting closer to sorting out the precarious road to treatment! It had been seven months since my toenail appointment.

The uncertainty was taking its toll on me and on Rob. We were protecting the kids from the details of my tests until we really knew what the long term prognosis would be. For the two of them, life was pretty normal except that, happily, their mom was home much more often these days. But Rob and I were living with the reality that not only was my life in jeopardy, our finances were also looking precarious as I was not working. Now we had to face the fact that I had many more months of interim treatment ahead just to possibly become well enough to undergo even more treatment.

The next mission, as I was popping steroids and healing my liver, was to finish the process of diagnosing the extent of the lymphoma. My oncologist was of the view that it was very slow-growing, and perhaps dormant, possibly lurking around for the past seven years. I was not so sure, so I sought a second opinion.

After duplicating a number of tests and reviewing my file, the second oncologist recommended a bone marrow biopsy to confirm staging. If the Hodgkin's is found in the bone marrow, this is not a good thing. But she said it was simply a confirmation of the staging she already suspected. The BMT was really only necessary to double check that it was not Stage IV (end stage). "Better safe than sorry" she said.

The bone marrow biopsy is another nasty procedure involving local anesthetic. Getting wise, I had read about it on the Internet before arriving, so this time I opted for the sedatives. I was feeling pretty good by the time two physicians showed up to conduct the procedure. They were young (very young, I thought), and arrived in a jocular mood. They apologized for keeping me waiting. It was so unusual to hear a physician apologize that I wondered in my jaded inside voice if they were rookies. The excuse they gave for being late was that they had had some difficulty with the prior patient, who had also had a bone marrow biopsy. Something to do with a "subcutaneous challenge" – at which they both sniggered. Knowing my medical terms by now, I quickly ascertained the nature of the problem: "you mean she was too fat?" This set them off into inappropriate peals of laughter.

I had lost ten pounds due to my liver issues, so I knew I was not subcutaneously challenged. I therefore expected my procedure to be less difficult for these two comedians. I misdiagnosed the situation. I only realized this after my pleasant morphine dream bubble was burst by a nasty, bone-jarring prod in my left pelvis.

"OUCH!" I said. "Sorry," they said. And then, to add insult to injury, they said they had not gotten enough marrow, and HAD TO DO IT AGAIN. Nothing worse. It was like someone banged a nail into my skeletal frame; my whole body reverberated with the impact. Twice.

Several weeks later, I received the desired second opinion on my cancer. Unfortunately, it was diametrically opposed to the first one. This second doctor pronounced that my Hodgkin's Disease was at Stage III and needed to be treated aggressively and quickly. The usual treatment for a relapse of this nature was extra high dosage chemotherapy; however, given my liver disorder, that was not recommended here. Instead, she suggested a hybrid chemo cocktail that was better tolerated by the liver. She did not volunteer the odds on this hybrid.

She then added to my frustration by letting me know that the results of the bone marrow biopsy turned out to be inconclusive – even the SECOND sample was insufficient! She did not believe the cancer had progressed to the bone marrow – meaning Stage IV –"or you would be a lot sicker", she said. But she still thought it was a good precautionary measure to have the procedure a third time.

My primary oncologist did not think it was necessary at all. His pragmatic rationale was that it would not change the course of my treatment as I was ineligible for the alternate treatment for Stage IV – a bone marrow transplant – due to my liver disease. Wham again.

I wanted to know anyway, so I submitted to a third attempt at this uncomfortable operation, perhaps just for the sake of having a test result that was good news for once.

As it turned out, this particular episode caused me more pain and anguish than anything else I had undertaken to that point. It was not the third procedure itself, which was thankfully uneventful and less painful this time, but the delivery of the results, which was emotionally traumatic.

Rumours of my demise

Several weeks after the third test, the report was sent to my oncologist. I went alone to this appointment as I did not expect more than a cursory confirmation of the good results.

I sat by myself in my oncologist's office and scanned the elusive biopsy report. My eyes moved laboriously over the medical jargon until I saw a heading "report results" and moved down the page to search for the expected words: "negative for bone marrow involvement". Instead, the bottom dropped out of my stomach, the blood left my head and I had to grab the arms of my chair as the reality of what was on the page dawned on me. "End stage … extensive musculoskeletal involvement … consistent with terminal disease".

What?? How could I have been so misled? How dare my doctor leave me here to read this alone? As I proceeded to go into total shock, something in the back of my brain nagged at me … something wasn't right. There was a word here that didn't compute … the report said "lung cancer". Surely it hadn't spread to my lungs, and from there to my bone marrow? There was no mention of lymphoma.

As I puzzled over this, I finally scanned back up to the top of the report, only to realize it was NOT MY NAME. Good God in heaven, they had given me the wrong report. This poor woman, Somebody McSomething, was dying of lung cancer, and I may actually have been one of the first people to know that.

As my heart pumped madly in my chest, I speculated about what would have happened if I had died of a massive coronary right there in the oncologist's office. Would my family be able to sue for something like "mistaken fatal diagnosis causing fatality"? Or would they ever know what had happened? Would anyone?

Call me chicken, I did not have the heart to point out the error to the overwhelmed oncologist. I quietly slipped the report back to the clerk who had delivered it, pointed to the name, and said "I don't think this is what you meant to give me." She blanched, and promptly located the right report, which proudly proclaimed "negative for bone marrow involvement" as we had all expected.

Phew. I had almost blocked the whole incident from my mind when I picked up the weekend newspaper several months later and sadly read the obituary of Mrs. McSomething. "In lieu of flowers, donations to the Canadian Lung Association gratefully accepted."

9

EXPLORING OTHER OPTIONS

Immediately following my visit to the enlightening hepatologist, I was started on a heavy dose of Prednisone. After a few weeks of steroidal mania during which I enjoyed manic insomnia, left kitchen burners on and dropped things a lot, my dosage was adjusted and I managed to avoid doing harm to myself or the general public. I turned my attention back to the job at hand: finding ways to take control of my healing.

One of the important possibilities for me to explore was the whole area of complementary healing alternatives such as nutrition, vitamins, supplements, naturopathic medicine, clinical trials, acupuncture, meditation, guided imagery, visualization, prayer, Reiki, reflexology – provided they were applied in an integrated way with my medical treatments. But the first time I inquired about pursuing these types of therapies, I was sternly warned about the dangers of any "alternative" treatment that was not medically proven. When I tried to explain that I wanted to explore these options in conjunction with, not instead of, my medical treatment, I was still not encouraged. My oncologist warned me about taking any homeopathic, herbal or vitamin remedies, for fear of drug interactions or liver effects. As for other options such as meditation, relaxation, massage, yoga, he said they couldn't hurt. He thought they might make me feel better, but did not seem to hold out any hope that they would contribute to a positive healing outcome.

In short, don't get your hopes up. But isn't that exactly what you want to do – get your hopes up?

Historically, the medical community has been taught only to prescribe treatment that has a body of scientific evidence supporting it. This attitude is slowly changing. Thankfully, the evidence supporting the healing effects of exercise, vitamins, diet and nutrition, meditation, yoga, Chi Qong and other therapies is starting to build.

Despite the warnings of the medical practitioners, I set out to find out more about integrative cancer care options. What I learned was ultimately, to me, life-saving information. I found out that many non-conventional therapies can boost your immune system to fight cancer and enhance your ability to tolerate treatments (chemotherapy, radiation and other invasive medical practices, such as surgery). Some may actually increase your response rate to conventional medical treatment, increasing your chances of survival.

I found that there are trained medical practitioners who will collaborate with your medical team to administer these complementary therapies, integrating them into the conventional treatment program to greatly enhance your ability to heal.

Healing mind, body and spirit

I did not know any of this before my journey was well under way in the conventional system. Initially, like many patients, I had accepted what I was being told about avoiding homeopathic remedies. But as part of my new take-charge treatment plan I decided to explore all of my options to heal – at all levels of mind, body and spirit, regardless of the potential resistance I might encounter.

The first step in my Heal Thyself project was to do some research. I read everything I could about my two diseases, about complementary healing options, about vitamins and supplements and possible interactions with chemotherapy drugs, effects on the liver, and so on. My research led me back to an organization where I had previously done some volunteer work: InspireHealth, a local centre for integrated cancer treatment. I had met with the CEO and board several years previously but had not expected I would later need their services as a patient.

I enrolled in their two-day Life Enhancing Seminar, now called the LIFE program. We were encouraged to bring a "caregiver", but Rob was not able to take time off work so Carol agreed to join me. By the time the workshop arrived, I was at a serious low point between treatments. I had constant chills and my lungs were so compromised that I could barely walk up a flight of stairs without gasping for breath. I thought about cancelling, but with Carol's encouragement I found the strength to get off the couch, get dressed and go.

The two-day seminar proved to be a transformative experience. On a practical level, I learned how to develop a customized program of exercise, nutrition, relaxation and self-care that I could adapt depending on how I was feeling. I learned about healing foods, therapeutic ingredients and supplements, and which toxic household products to banish from my cupboards. I learned visualization techniques I could use to encourage my body to fight the cancer cells.

At a more profound level, I learned about mental and spiritual aspects of healing, which are rarely addressed by conventional medical practitioners. We were taught about the "Top 11" attributes of patients who had experienced remission in the face of a terminal diagnosis. In many ways, this could be called a recipe for how to live one's life. With credit to the dedicated team at InspireHealth, I have included the list below.

"The majority of people who recover from advanced 'incurable' cancer exhibit many or all of the following characteristics:

1.   They have a deep belief in their body's ability to heal in spite of being told by their doctor that their illness is terminal.

2. They regain a sense of control in their lives – a feeling that they can substantially impact their own health and healing. They assume responsibility for creating a recovery program that is right for them – they do not simply abdicate responsibility for their treatment to their doctor.

3. They undergo a "spiritual transformation" – an awakening of the true values and aspirations that had lain dormant inside them. Truly alive – perhaps for the first time – this spiritual re-awakening brings a new authenticity to their life as they reconnect with their deepest values and aspirations. Once healed, they may look back upon their illness as a "gift" that helped transform their life.

4. They bring a new authenticity to their relationships with others and the world around them.

5. They fully reassess their lives – often making very significant changes to their diet, lifestyle, career, goals, and relationships with others.

6. They often make radically healthful changes in their diet – away from refined, processed foods towards healthful, wholesome foods. They eat more fruits and vegetables and less animal fat, and many become vegetarian.

7. They take vitamins and supplements to help support their health and immune system.

8. They take more time to simply relax and enjoy their life. For many, meditation or prayer becomes an important part of their daily life.

9. They learn to 'listen' to their bodies and to surrender to, rather than resist, the day-to-day fluctuations of energy, symptoms and emotions that accompany the healing process. In doing so, they listen to their bodies for guidance for optimally loving and taking care of themselves.

10. They release any sense of guilt about fully caring for themselves. In so doing, they learn to fully love and support themselves – creating a wonderful life that optimally supports health.

11. They reconnect with their sense of community and reclaim the joy that comes from being of service to others. In healing themselves, they facilitate healing in others."

Source: www.inspirehealth.ca

This list resonated with me because it validated many of the practices I had already been pursuing by hit or miss. It gave me the encouragement to maintain my basic health and diet regime while embarking on a parallel course of self-discovery, changes in lifestyle, spiritual exploration and finding new ways to be of service to others.

The power of the mind

One of the "aha" moments in the seminar for me occurred during a guided visualization. One of the centre's practitioners took us through a deep relaxation exercise, and then guided us on an imagined journey. We were invited to see ourselves resting in bed, then getting out of bed and making our way to the kitchen. We were encouraged to feel the carpet or bare floor with the soles of our feet as we walked to the refrigerator. As we opened the fridge, we felt the cold blast of air raising goose bumps on our flesh; we reached into the fridge and brought out a lemon. We felt the cold, dimpled skin of the firm lemon in our hand. We located a sharp knife and a cutting board, and sliced the lemon in four pieces. We were then invited to take one of the quarters and put it to our mouth, biting into the tart fruit.

After she brought us back to a fully awake state, she asked us if we had noticed anything during the visioning session. I said, "My saliva glands went crazy when I bit the lemon." Yes, she said, how many had that experience? Everyone had.

She then reminded us that "there was no lemon. What was it that made your saliva glands activate, then?" Clearly, it was our minds.

"Yes, and if the mind can do that, would you also believe it can activate healing processes throughout your body?"

It would be hard to argue otherwise, yet most of us are not educated to believe in "thinking ourselves well". It smacks of faith healing or telekinesis. Yet here was clear evidence that thoughts can influence bodily functions. I determined from that point on to practice visualization as part of my healing regimen.

The path to self-discovery

The InspireHealth seminar also provided a gentle invitation for those who felt the inspiration to do some spiritual work as part of our healing journey. Some of my fellow seminar attendees chose to accept the invitation; some didn't. I was game, but not quite sure where to begin.

I found some answers when I had my first one-to-one consultation with InspireHealth CEO Dr. Hal Gunn, a man who views integrated cancer care as his life's calling. He is a gifted and insightful specialist, with an incredible knowledge of research and treatment, and a passion for finding new ways of preventing cancer, enhancing recovery rates and reducing recurrence.

Dr. Gunn encouraged me to follow a consistent program of nutrition, sleep, yoga, meditation and visualization, and continued exercise (walking, whatever I felt up to, as long as I did it consistently — even when my treatments made me feel like the last thing I wanted to do was get off the couch). He also recommended a fortifying combination of vitamins and an immune boosting supplement to accelerate my response to chemotherapy, minimize damaging side effects, heal my liver, and generally improve my overall feeling of well-being. Dr. Gunn conferred with my medical specialists to ensure my regime was integrated and complementary to my other treatments.

Suddenly, I felt empowered and truly equipped to take control of making myself well. It was a liberating realization. Armed with this integrated conventional and complementary care regime, I felt I had already radically improved the odds of achieving my "Project: Heal Kathy McLaughlin" goal.

But Dr. Gunn was not finished with me yet. In my next session with him, he had asked me if I thought there were emotional or spiritual questions I wanted to explore. He invited me, with a very gentle nudge, to examine this a little further. He sensed that I already knew what I had to do. His contribution, simply through his steady soul-penetrating gaze, was to confirm my commitment to doing it.

Following that visit, I set out on a deeper self-discovery path. Once again, I consciously decided to create a structured project plan for my psycho-spiritual journey. I knew it was a life and death matter and I needed to impose some self-discipline to stick to my intentions.

Ultimately, I embarked on three areas of focus:

- *Radical self-care*: adopting much more responsible and consistent health habits including nutrition, exercise, vitamins, relaxation, meditation, me-time, self-rewards and lots and lots of sleep.
- *Making peace*: laying down my weapons. Learning how to curb my anger, heal my relationships, practice self-forgiveness and forgiveness of others. Finding keys to unlock my heart and connect with others on an intimate level.
- *Exploring my purpose*: finding ways to align my work with my heart.

I mapped out some action steps, which included making several appointments: first, with a psychotherapist; second, a spiritual advisor; and third, a newly-trained Reiki specialist, Ruth, a friend who kindly volunteered her services to help practice her new skill. In addition, my mother arranged for me to have reflexology treatments, and bought us both tickets to attend a future workshop with Adam McLeod, a young phenomenon who had authored a series of books about energy healing (www.dreamhealer.com).

Reaching out to a guru

Several months into my journey of self-discovery, I did something rather impulsively, perhaps guided by intuition. I called the office of Dr. Gabor Maté, a locally renowned physician and author of several inspired books. A friend with cancer had given me his first book, *When the Body Says No*. It talks about the family roots of disease (both hereditary and psycho-spiritual). Dr. Maté expresses his view that cancer and other diseases are related to the need to heal the heart and psyche, and that the physical disease is simply a symptom, or clue, of deep-seated distress.

I was put through to Dr. Maté's voice messaging box, where in a rather brusque voice he stated his inability to take on new patients at present. I realized that just leaving a name and number would not be the best way to get a response. So I blurted the executive summary of my story onto his voicemail, in a rapid and breathless monologue. "Hello, Dr. Maté, you don't know me and I know you're not seeing new patients, but I have read all of your books and would be very grateful if I could see you for a short visit to get your advice on my situation. I have had cancer twice, and also have end stage liver disease, theoretically unrelated. I am on a journey to discover the work I need to do to heal my heart, body and soul once and for all." Perhaps a rather bold and candid message to leave for a complete stranger, I thought. But what did I have to lose? My mind told me he would be too busy to return the call; my heart told me otherwise.

He called within twenty-four hours, encountering my voice mail, and simply said I should call his office to make an appointment. I did so, and got the man himself rather than his voice mail this time. "Can you come in next Tuesday at 1 p.m.?" Miraculous. That was one of the moments in my life that cemented my belief that little miracles can happen as long as we put ourselves in their path.

Dr. Maté asked me similar questions as had Dr. Gunn, but with a more clinical manner. He did not lack warmth – clearly his life has been devoted to compassionate work – but he was amazingly efficient at asking tough questions: "What do you want?"; "Why do you think that?"; "How do you know that is true?"; "Is this a story you are telling, or do you know it is a fact?"

After listening intensely, the wise Dr. Maté prescribed four steps for me:

- Reading *"Loving What Is"* by Byron Katie and Stephen Mitchell (Three Rivers Press, New York, 2002)
- Meditation
- Body work with a gifted healer he recommended
- Attending a workshop on self-discovery – he recommended several in the local vicinity.

I had some important coordinates to help me navigate through the spiritual leg of my journey.

10

From Near Death to New Life

Meanwhile, miraculously, my liver started to respond to the steroids. And my new integrated health regime seemed to be helping my body fight for itself. My enzyme levels were improving and some of the worst symptoms of liver failure, such as abdominal swelling and jaundice, were under control.

My oncologist had consulted with the BC Cancer Agency to come up with an experimental chemotherapy regime that was easier on the liver than the conventional treatment. While there were no guarantees, the doctors felt that this was the only hope to fight my cancer without destroying my liver.

After four months of steady improvement, I was pronounced ready to tolerate this new assault on my system. My compassionate oncologist wanted to postpone things until after Christmas, really for no reason other than to allow me to enjoy the holiday season. But I wanted to get on with it NOW, lest I somehow miss the window of opportunity. I pleasantly and persistently won him over. My treatment regime was expected to last six or seven months.

This coincided nicely with the timing for an executive coaching course I had enrolled in. Even before my diagnosis I had known I wanted to move my career in a new direction. Becoming an executive coach seemed like a perfect way to answer my desire to help people, while capitalizing on my corporate career and executive search background. I viewed it as a bit of synchronicity that the course dates exactly paralleled the period of time I would be undergoing chemotherapy. I could learn a new vocation and get my mind off the grueling challenge ahead. I visualized attending my graduation ceremony cancer-free – new and improved!

I expected to sail through chemo as efficiently as I had done the first time around. At first, everything seemed familiar. My hair fell out right on schedule – this time it was the week the Pope died. During my first traumatic encounter with total hair loss, the world had lost Princess Diana. This time, Pope John Paul II decided to check out. I can't explain why my hair decided to fall out at the exact times that two famous personages met their demise, but to me both events were a poignant reminder of the triviality of my vanity against the inescapable reality of death. As if to reinforce my personal quest, these were the deaths of two people who had devoted their lives to being in service of others.

Rather than hide from reality this time, I proudly sent bald photos of myself to my cadre of followers. I felt like it was important to go public with my reality, not to disguise my truth under wigs, hats or bandannas. This was more to acknowledge that I was on a different path than to seek sympathy. For years I had been wearing costumes and playing roles on a self-conceived stage where falling ill would have been a fatal admission of weakness. I wanted to embrace my reality, rather than pretend everything was someone else's definition of normal.

Years later, my feelings were echoed in a cathartic *Sex and the City* episode where Samantha, undergoing cancer treatment, speaks at a breast cancer benefit. After valiantly trying to maintain her composure and pretend she is not suffering all of the unpleasant side effects of chemo, she starts to visibly melt from a combined hot flash and the sauna of her wig. People start to shift their eyes and look embarrassed for her (a look I knew all too well). In disgust, she finally dispenses with the façade, declares "F--- it!", and wrenches her scratchy, sweaty synthetic coif from her relieved, and very bald, scalp. Women across the room stand up in silent solidarity, flinging off their own wigs to reveal themselves as beautifully bald, courageous fighters. Samantha ceremoniously twirls the offending hairpiece high above the crowd and then launches it permanently into outer space, to cheers and a standing ovation.

A close call

After an easy beginning, my chemo treatments proved to be much more brutal this time around. Following the third treatment, I was decidedly weak and nauseous, glued to the couch and clearly not much help around the house. Then my temperature started to climb. It was still not in the danger zone by evening, so Rob and I decided to go to bed and check it in the morning.

By morning it was still hovering on the fringe of the danger zone, but had not climbed. We decided Rob should take Maddie to her volleyball game while I rested at home with my cell phone handy. Rob would leave his on too, in case I needed to call.

I fell asleep immediately, but awoke in an hour feeling hot and sweaty. I reached for the thermometer and waited as it shot up – 102F. Danger zone! I grabbed the cell phone and dialed Rob's number, only to receive the annoying automated voice: "The customer you are calling is currently unavailable. Please try your call again later." There was no cell coverage at the gym!

Somewhat panicky, I started calling my neighbours to see if they could take me to Emergency. No one home. My sister was out. My mother was out. Even my dad and stepmom were out. Unbelievably, no one could be reached. I tried Rob again. Still unavailable. I took my temperature again – 104F! Now really alarmed, I tried Rob's number about five more times, not really thinking productively about who else I could call.

Finally, as my temperature hovered around 105F, Rob and Maddie returned from the game. Rob quickly made his way to the laundry room, out of earshot from the family room where I lay weakly waiting to be rescued. So my first hysterical yell of "why didn't you answer my calls, we have to go to the hospital!" did not get Rob's attention. Maddie came running in and realized that her mother was in serious trouble, and we both tried to get through to Rob that it was time to go to the hospital. Incredibly, he was still unable to hear over the roar of the washing machine as he proceeded to put on a load of laundry and tidy the kitchen.

When we arrived at Emergency I was nearly unconscious. Rob quickly explained my history and symptoms to the triage nurse. I was immediately whisked into an isolation room and hooked up to an IV for a mega dose of antibiotics. The ER doctor chastised both of us for waiting so long to get here. My temperature was now above 105F, close to a life-threatening level. The doctor seemed genuinely worried that he would not be able to arrest the infection before I went into septic shock.

Luckily, I responded quickly to the antibiotics. To be on the safe side, the doctors wanted to keep me on the IV for at least four days; I was admitted to an upstairs ward to lie in bed for a long, slow drip.

A little miracle

That evening Rob brought Maddie and Conor in to see me. I felt frustrated and sad that I had to stay here instead of tucking them into their beds. Maddie had brought me her favourite stuffed animal, a well-loved blue and white dog named Ellen, who had accompanied her on many sleepovers and family vacation adventures. Ellen's music box used to play the Lullaby song. It was both kids' favorite as babies when I sang them to sleep. The strains of that song seemed to be reassuring, healing even, and it had almost always calmed both babies when nothing else worked. Sadly, Ellen's music box no longer played; but Ellen herself didn't seem to mind. She continued looking at us lovingly with her dark glass puppy-eyes. Maddie had brought Ellen to keep me company. In my fragile state, this little gesture brought tears to my eyes.

I was still crying when they all left, but tried to hide it so the kids wouldn't be alarmed. I felt so alone and lonely in the hospital room, and still a little scared that the infection could flare up again. It was the first time I had felt this close to the possibility that cancer – or treatment – could claim me.

I fiddled with Ellen's wind up key, and said a little prayer for her mechanism to be fixed so I could hear the Lullaby song one more time. No such luck.

To get my mind off things, I turned on the TV and started to get involved in a light, made-for-TV movie. About twenty minutes later a commercial came on. It was a car ad – for Honda, I think. A driverless car was pulling up to a toll booth. The car was obviously not able to pay the toll, and the toll booth operator was getting annoyed. Then the car turned its radio on and played a song. This promptly soothed the watchman to sleep, and the car drove on. Unbelievably, the song the car had played was – the Lullaby song!

Call it a coincidence … I believed it was a little miracle. It made me feel a lot better, and I thanked the universe for my reassuring message.

The big miracle

I reached the half-way mark in my treatments, and learned the bad news that my oncologist was not happy with my progress. He was now recommending a much higher dose of chemotherapy. He explained that there was a risk to my liver if he increased the dosage, but there was a bigger risk that the cancer would not respond if he didn't. We agreed to proceed.

Several days after that treatment, I experienced excruciating pain in my abdomen. There was blood in my stool. I went back to the oncologist, only to learn that the chemo had burned the lining of my stomach, causing an ulcer. He prescribed morphine for the pain and Losec™ for the ulcer, and advised me it would heal slowly.

He was forced to go back to a slightly lower dose of chemo in the hopes that we could find a happy medium.

These and other setbacks resulted in delays to my treatment schedule. By the time my executive coaching graduation approached, I was only three-quarters of the way through chemo. I was weak, bald and uncertain about the future. However, I was very proud to have finished the program, and despite my doctor's admonition to avoid travel, I decided to make the trek to Victoria to attend my final capstone panel and the wrap-up ceremony. Despite my frail state, I passed the capstone - an intimidating coaching demonstration in front of a panel of judges and a room full of people. My colleagues all knew what I had been going through and cheered loudly as I was presented with my graduate certificate as a Certified Executive Coach.

I finished my treatments four months later. I will never forget the day I sat at the oncologist's office, waiting my turn to be ushered into the examining room. When the doctor emerged from a previous patient, he caught sight of me in the waiting room. His face broke into a huge grin, and he walked right over to me, shook my hand and patted me on the shoulder. "Go right in," he said, as if he could hardly wait to talk to me. In the privacy of the examination room he advised me there were no signs of tumours or even shadows on my PET and CT scans!

"We got lucky," he said. "Mission Impossible accomplished." I did not realize until that moment that he had truly thought our mission was impossible! He went on to say he thought I had been the beneficiary of a miracle. I thought he was being modest, and gave him much of the credit for figuring out the right treatment regime and persisting when it got dicey. He put a hand around my shoulders and simply said, "No, it was all you," and pointed to my head.

It was an important moment for me, as I realized that this very wise, deeply experienced medical doctor was crediting my positive attitude as the deciding factor in my healing.

Searching for a new path

The cancer battle was finally behind me! The matter of my ailing liver still lurked in the background, but I was determined to do everything I could to fortify what was left of it and perhaps defy the odds again. I vowed to continue my healing practices and to incorporate the learning from my spiritual and emotional exploration into a more balanced and grounded lifestyle.

I enjoyed a sunny month of recuperation during August, when Vancouver was at its best, and spent another week at Savary Island to enjoy my family.

I went back to work at the executive search firm in September, and was incredibly grateful to be warmly welcomed back by my partners. But I felt like a fickle lover. My newfound love of coaching distracted me from my former dedication to building a search practice. I tried to establish a coaching practice at the firm and at first my partners were very supportive. But the metrics just did not work in a business that was focused on retained search as its core competency. Coaching contracts were by nature lower in dollar volume, and I realized that to carry my weight, I needed to continue to bring in new search assignments. Eventually the coaching had to take a back seat as my workload mounted. By Christmas I was back to working sixteen-hour days on search assignments, trying to squeeze coaching sessions between interviews, and not really doing justice to either.

I knew I could not let myself fall back into the trap of working too hard and losing sight of my passion. Just as I was thinking about how to transition to an environment that was more aligned with my purpose, as if to answer my intention, I was fortunate to be offered a role as VP with a locally based manufacturer of soft leather baby shoes, Robeez Footwear Inc. This bright little gem of a company had been created by a woman entrepreneur, Sandra Wilson, and had gone viral to be THE brand of choice for early infant footwear in North America, the UK, Europe and Australia. Celebrities were spotted wearing Robeez on the red carpet. It was the designer baby's choice of accessory! The company had an excellent product, happy customers and a happy work culture. The new CEO had been recruited from Disney and had an exciting mandate to take the company to the next level. When he offered me the role of VP of Marketing I quickly accepted, and found myself in a position where I could mentor smart young marketing and sales people to promote wonderful merchandise. I loved my boss, the owners and my peers, and enjoyed the eager team that reported to me. It was an inspiring culture that allowed me to make use of my sales, marketing and leadership experience while also applying my coaching skills.

It was all of that for the first five months. I knew when I joined that Sandra was looking for partners to help her to transition out of being in the business full time. In fact, those of us who had joined the new leadership team were hoping to be able to take an equity position as we helped to grow the company. But as luck would have it, Sandra received an offer that she ultimately could not refuse, from Stride-Rite Shoes, a large corporate shoe company out of Boston. They bought the whole company. Over time things changed, and for me, it started to feel like a bad case of déjà vu. I found myself reporting to a remote head office run by tough-minded West Point grads who managed everything by the numbers. They were smart and savvy, but ultimately their role was to integrate the perky, independent Robeez culture into the large corporate process of their world. The CEO who had hired me left the company, and my new boss arrived from L.A. the next day. He had a marketing background, so it was clear fairly early on that one of us was redundant. He offered me a sales management role that would have involved a lot of travel. This was shaping up to look a lot like the worst parts of the corporate roles I thought I had left behind, and I started to feel an all-too- familiar psychic pain and panic.

Unable to see a logical way out, I consulted my own coach, one of my coaching school instructors. She reminded me to "listen to my heart". She also wisely pointed out that I was in the driver's seat. I had a healthy out-clause in my contract, and did not need to accept the definition of the new role the company was offering me. It was a liberating conversation, and ultimately I chose to request a severance package rather than stay on in the new role.

I agreed to stay through year-end and was amicably paid out, giving me enough of a cushion to start my own coaching and consulting business. I made the exhilarating leap! In many ways, the unexpected turn of events was the best thing that could have happened to me.

March 1996:
Selected as a 40 under
40 high achiever. The
future looked rosy!

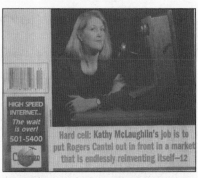

September 1996:
My 40th birthday,
before all the trouble.
My staff at Cantel
raided the promo
balloon supply.

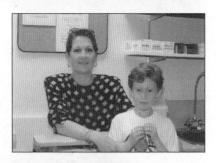

April 1997:
Diagnosed. Conor,
always Mr. Curiosity,
came with me to my
first chemo appoint-
ment. Now he works
in that hospital.

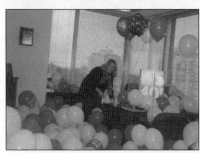

October 1997:
the chemo did what
it was supposed to.
Earrings helped.

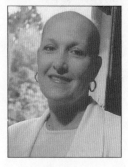

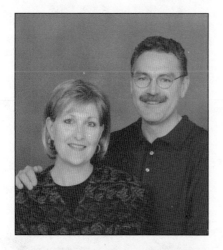

1998:
Wash n' wear synthetic
bob! Some days I
still wish I had it.

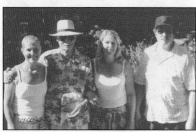

Spring 1998:
with Dad, sis and
bro. For several years,
no one mistook
me for Carol.

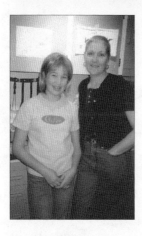

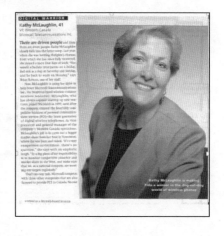

Wig swapping with
niece Charlotte. She
wanted to keep it.

1998:
Cancer well behind me, new hair; Canadian
Press describes me as a "driven" executive.

2004: Back to normal: one of our treasured summers at Savary with kids

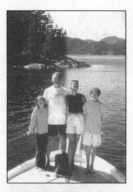

2006: celebrated my 50th and return to full health (so I thought) with a Hawaii 5-0 party.

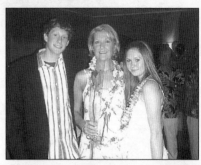

2007- 9: frequent customer at Vancouver General. Maddie brought me her stuffed dog "Ellen" for comfort.

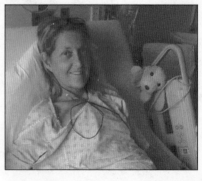

2012: doctors and media call me a miracle

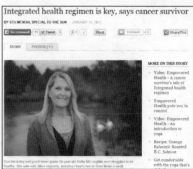

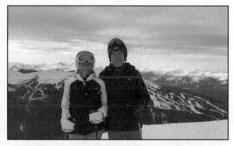

No one thought I would ski again. So I did. (Whistler, BC)

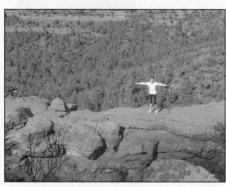

Many more mountains to climb (Devil's Bridge, Sedona)

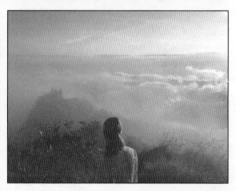

On top of the world (Mt. Batur, Bali, at dawn)

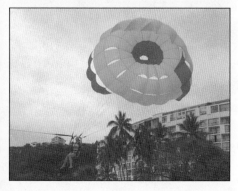

Embracing life from a new vantage point.

11

Not So Fast!

My consulting business took off pretty much from the beginning. I started by letting a few people know I was now certified as an executive coach, and those assignments led to additional work in the areas of organizational development and strategic planning. Seventeen years in telecom and four years in executive search had enabled me to build a strong business network. I started to get referrals from current and former clients, and was thoroughly enjoying the variety of my new assignments. I considered myself extremely lucky that I was able to work from a home office, and had the flexibility to spend time with the kids, make a good living, but also take time off if I was feeling tired or coping with the symptoms of my liver disease. Many of my clients did not even know about my medical history or liver condition.

For the better part of the next two years I enjoyed relatively good health. I saw my oncologist every six months, and he was convinced I was in complete remission. My liver enzymes had been stable, so the gastroenterologist, my GP and I all thought I was in pretty darn good shape for someone who had been through cancer and chemo twice, and had about twenty-five per cent of a liver left. I was mostly functioning like a normal healthy person, and by all accounts I looked great. My doctors continually told me that I looked unusually robust for someone "in my condition".

It is possible to carry on a pretty normal life with a fraction of a liver, provided it does not further deteriorate. Most of the time, with a little effort, I managed to put in the working mom-of-teens routine, work full time, buy groceries, make dinner, help the kids with their homework, drive Maddie to soccer and Conor to his part-time jobs. Laden still came back to clean our house and visit every week or two. In between, Rob did more than his share of laundry, dishes, vacuuming and grocery shopping. The kids occasionally pitched in when fatigue got the better of me, but I rarely played the "sick mom" card.

Admittedly, there were a number of symptoms that I was learning to work around. In the overall scheme of things, compared with what I had been through, I easily relegated them to the category of minor aggravations. These included an inability to drink even one glass of my favorite Chardonnay without a hangover. So, I confined my wine enjoyment to a thimbleful of a really great vintage now and then, and smugly congratulated myself the next morning when the rest of the partygoers were nursing headaches.

Another annoyance was my protruding abdomen. The size of the pot belly seemed to fluctuate, but when it was bad, I looked eight months pregnant and could not eat more than a few mouthfuls of anything without feeling full. I was retaining anywhere from 10 to 15 lbs of water, but had lost body fat and muscle mass everywhere else. No butt, no boobs, no flaps, no love handles; just stick-thin arms and legs and a bloated belly with an Etch-a-Sketch pattern of surgery scars.

Running downhill

I was also finding it challenging to maintain my fitness routine. Most frustratingly, it seemed I would never be able to return to running, due to reduced lung capacity. In the back of my mind I still thought of myself as a runner. A year after my last chemo treatment I had worked my way back up to jog-walking the seawall. I had often passed my oncologist and his wife on their evening walk. I thought this was particularly appropriate as it allowed him to appreciate the after-effects of one of his many "miracles". However, to my dismay, there seemed to be fewer and fewer days when my lungs were clear enough to jog, and some days it was hard even to get up a flight of stairs or the driveway without gasping for air.

Initially I had attributed this to chemo damage. At the end of my first round of cancer treatments, I had lost thirty per cent of my lung capacity and was told the damage was permanent. At the end of round two, I never bothered to have a pulmonary function test since I guessed it would simply tell me even worse news. To add insult to injury, I was required to wear a medic alert necklace identifying my lung damage in case I needed oxygen for some reason, as I was told my lungs could "blow up". I had visions of accidentally exploding at the hands of an unwitting paramedic. Ironically, I felt like I needed oxygen on a daily basis.

I finally went back to see my gastroenterologist to see if he could determine why my air capacity was getting progressively worse. After a barrage of tests (CT, X-ray, ultrasound), he identified the problem as "pleural effusion" (fluid above the diaphragm) combined with "ascites" (fluid below the diaphragm). Basically my lungs were surrounded by water. This was not an unusual by-product of a sick liver. As the fluid increased, my lungs were slowly collapsing.

The key to removing this internal water balloon was to increase my dosage of diuretics. However, that produced frustrating side effects including nightly muscle spasms that progressed from my toes to my feet, legs, hands and eventually both of my hamstrings (really painful!). I spent many a night dancing, cursing and howling at the moon, which seems quite funny in retrospect but was not very amusing at the time.

In addition to dancing by night, I was running by day, so to speak. For the year and a half since my chemo treatments had ended, I had lived with a bad case of "unpredictable bowel syndrome". I was losing a lot of weight, as it seemed that anything I ingested left in a real hurry, often pretty much intact. (Too much information, sorry.) This tended to be very awkward if I was conducting a workshop with a room full of executives. I invented clever new "pop quizzes" and team exercises to manufacture unscheduled breaks when needed.

The symptoms I was experiencing were all common indications of late stage cirrhosis. The treatment was to stabilize the symptoms with drugs and other interventions, continue on steroids and a restricted diet to ensure the liver did not sustain further damage, and "carry on".

Uncle, really!

Using what I had learned through my integrated cancer healing program, I continued with my extra healthy diet, took my vitamins, exercised when I could, and quietly coped with the annoyances. Most of all, I worked on maintaining my optimism and acting as normal as I could, with the cheerful assumption that all would be well. I continued to go after new client assignments, attend meetings and dress the part even on days when I felt like going back to bed. While I did not feel like I was pushing myself too hard, I did feel that a normal work load was getting harder and harder to endure due to fatigue and the cumulative effect of an increasing number of ailments.

The area where I cut corners, as always when "real work" presented itself, was at home. Given my odd diet and state of exhaustion, I was not always good at putting dinner on the table. Rob and the kids ate a lot of Kraft Dinner in that era, though Rob often pitched in with his killer spaghetti, or take-out deli specials. Things were in an adjusted holding pattern, a suspended state of near-health that I felt I could endure for a long time. Some days, I even felt like my liver might be improving, and continued to do my meditation, visualization and self-grounding to give myself the best chance of healing.

Nonetheless, over the course of the next year, my symptoms got progressively worse, including severe gastric pain. It was as if I had food poisoning every other day or so. After six months of chronic burning, aching, diarrhea and further weight loss, I went from enjoying my new-normal life to serious frustration that I could not seem to stabilize this leaky vessel after the long storm. One night, in sheer frustration, I composed an email to my gastroenterologist detailing my increasingly serious complaints:

Dear Doctor:

I thought I would set out my current symptoms in a message before I come in to see you, in case it helps to decipher what is going on:

Frequent abdominal pain, left lower side, kidneys, radiating to upper right side, area of gallbladder. Some sharp pains, mostly ongoing dull chronic ache from stomach down to lower organs. This has been going on for more than four months intermittently, and without relief for the past 4-5 days.

Continued ascites, not responding to diuretics. At peak, you can hear my abdomen sloshing loudly when I walk.

Headache, chills but no fever.

Dizziness.

Chronic diarrhea, alternating with light coloured, frequent soft stool; painful elimination (lower abdominal cramping).

Extreme shortness of breath, inability to walk up my driveway or resume normal exercise routine.

Extreme fatigue, early morning and late afternoon.

Bleeding gums, nasal passages.

Frequent coughing and gagging, difficulty swallowing, blockage in throat.

Weight and muscle mass loss – approx. 20 lbs, mostly from arms and legs (certainly not abdomen!). Weight fluctuates from 162 when ascites is at peak, to 137.0 – 10 lbs below normal weight. Extreme muscle cramps in legs and feet, every hour or so at night; cramps in fingers and hands throughout the day.

Muscle aches in shoulder / neck area.

Ringing in the ears.

No visible signs of jaundice.

Insomnia, resulting in obsessive late-night emails to medical professionals (☺).

This got his attention. More accurately it got his assistant's attention. She said it had made her "very sad" and she had put it right in front of him. I thought perhaps I had overreacted to get his attention, and now she thought I was dying.

Maybe he did, too, because very quickly, after thinking the storm was behind me, I was plunged once again into the eye of the hurricane with CT scans, colonoscopies, gastroscopies, a pleural paracentesis, blood tests and weekly diagnostic visits to the gastroenterologist. After weeks of procedures, the doctor was still totally stumped. He doubled my diuretics to try to make a real dent in the fluid retention, hoping the pain would also be resolved. My water levels did decline, to the point that I lost six more pounds. My arms and legs were really scrawny.

In the midst of all of this, I was approached by a head hunter for a CEO role I found very attractive. It was in the field of cancer fundraising, and was one of the few corporate roles for which I would have considered giving up my consulting practice. My fear was whether we would solve this medical conundrum in time for me to regain the energy to jump back into such a demanding job. The thought of early morning breakfast meetings, corporate dinner meetings, frequent travel and meeting the needs of a staff of one hundred seemed completely out of the question for me right now. Still, ever the optimist, I pulled myself together and made it through several interviews. Thankfully, the state of my health was not obvious to the search committee, and I was ultimately shortlisted as one of two finalist candidates.

As I was waiting to hear the final outcome and worrying about whether I had any business thinking I could tackle such a significant role, my symptoms started to worsen.

I experienced gastric pain so intense that I wondered if it was an ulcer from obsessing over the potential responsibility of the job. I called the doctor and he sent me to Emergency to get a fresh assessment of my symptoms.

After six hours of tests, the ER doctors could not pinpoint the problem but ruled out infection and dubbed it gastritis – "inflammation of the gastric tract". *Ha*, I thought, *I could have told them that!* They advised me to take medication usually prescribed for people with ulcers or colitis. I wondered if they were thinking it was a "nervous stomach" or something similarly psychosomatic. As I had suspected, perhaps this was just a side effect of agonizing over my career decision.

But when the doctor saw me the following Monday he reminded me this symptom had plagued me off and on for several months. He believed it was more than a worried stomach: he suspected bile duct blockage or gallstones and wanted to order a camera scope to have a good look through the lower abdominal tract. He also wanted to biopsy the small bowel as there was some discernible "thickening" that could be inflammation. He did not say so at the time, but by the look on his face I wondered if he suspected that my cancer had found a new location to invade.

I left his office feeling much more worried than when I arrived, facing the bleak prospect of more scopes and scans. If we didn't figure things out soon, I would be crazy to consider a career change – or any career at all.

Despite this gloomy thought, I thanked the doctor for all of his diligent investigation on my behalf, and we wished each other a good week.

The next morning, all hell broke loose. I just didn't know it.

My lost day

My day started with Conor saying a hasty goodbye to me as I lay on the couch in the family room. I had apparently neglected to wake the kids for school. Conor had managed to lurch out of bed "just in time", and thoughtfully yelled some choice expletives to wake up his sister. On their way out the door they discovered me semi-comatose on the couch, and said goodbye. I mumbled and waved groggily. Neither of the kids thought my behaviour unusual enough to be concerned, even though my normal routine on a work day would be to get up at 6 a.m., do my email, organize my day and make several phone calls before waking the kids, making them breakfast and driving them to school. Normal for me was *not* sleeping on the couch until noon.

Sometime after noon a delivery man came to the door with a package for Rob. His loud knocking roused me from my stupor. I was able to get to the door but was not very helpful to the poor man. I remember thinking vaguely that he must have the wrong house because he obviously didn't speak my language. After trying to understand what he was saying, I waved an unsteady "talk to the hand" gesture, slammed the door on him in mid-sentence and retreated back to the comfort of my couch. Intent on completing his mission, the delivery man called Rob's office to explain that he had tried to make his delivery and get a signature for the parcel, but "the lady at the door didn't speak English."

Rob did not get that message because he was already on his way home to check on the delivery. He caught the frustrated messenger in the driveway just in time to sign for the package. The man did not repeat his story about a failed attempt to deliver because he thought Rob had gotten the message. Rob came in the house, found me on the couch, but did not think that too unusual as sometimes I did take cat naps. I gave him a rather unintelligible response to his greeting, but he thought I was just tired, and he returned to work.

When he got back to the office his assistant advised him of the strange message. Finally realizing that something was wrong, he rushed home to find me awake but incoherent. I had 'come to' around 3 p.m. and by the time Rob arrived, I was in a state of panic, trying to remember how to dial my cell phone. I could not remember any phone numbers or how to access the directory. I could not even read the numbers. I had tried to walk to the kitchen to find a phone book, but my legs had been so wobbly it felt like I was on the moon. I had given up and crumpled into a cross-legged heap on the floor, which is where Rob found me, staring at the wall, mumbling "something's wrong, something's wrong". He quickly rounded up the kids and packed me off to Emergency for the second time in a week.

By the time we arrived, I had regained control of some of my faculties. I valiantly tried to behave as if everything was normal. I was proudly able to remember my long list of prescription drugs. It did seem I was improving. However, when asked the standard question about any allergies, I quite matter-of-factly slurred that I was "allergic to surgery". This prompted the triage nurse to ask Rob if I had spent the day cleaning out our liquor cabinet.

An inconvenient patient

When the Admitting nurse finally ascertained that I was a legitimate sick person suffering from end stage liver disease, things started to happen very quickly. I was rushed into a private room in Emergency and hooked up to what seemed like every piece of equipment they could find. Given my symptoms, the doctors suspected I was suffering from a build-up of ammonia that is a common side effect of liver failure, which can be fatal if not treated immediately. Known as hepatic encephalopathy, the condition is defined in Wikipedia as *"the occurrence of confusion, altered level of consciousness, and coma as a result of liver failure. In the advanced stages it is called hepatic coma or coma hepaticum. It may ultimately lead to death"*.

This explained why I felt so gooned. At the time, I did not realize it was that serious, and I was so punch-drunk that I found everything rather entertaining. I thought myself quite witty as I prattled away at Rob and anyone else who would listen.

My family and I now think back on the story of my "lost day" with some amusement. Whenever I act silly, Conor gives me "the look" and says, "Should we call someone?"

However, at the time it just served to underscore the reality of my severely worsening condition. Clearly my liver was deteriorating at a rapid rate. I was worried, Rob was worried, and all of my doctors were worried.

Don't make any long-term plans

The day after I was released from hospital, I received a call from the headhunter advising me that the other finalist had been chosen for the CEO role. Given the circumstances, I was highly relieved. I most certainly would have had to turn down the opportunity if it had gone the other way, with a lot of guilt and regret. Instead, I took this as a rather clear message to dedicate my energy to healing.

At this stage the doctor enlisted the help of the BC Transplant team to conduct a full appraisal of my liver condition and assess my eligibility for a transplant. The Transplant team ordered another barrage of tests, including a CT scan, ultrasound, X-rays, pulmonary function test, respiratory consultation, various urine and blood tests, a TB test, a mammogram and an MRI. I spent two more months getting poked, prodded and squeezed in aid of determining whether I was at the stage where I should be put on the transplant waiting list.

Coordinating the schedule for all of this was a full-time job in itself. I had to do things in a certain sequence or they would create problems for other procedures. Since two different sources were requesting the tests, it was pretty much up to me to mediate this. In one particular week, I had the pulmonary function test, mammogram, X-ray and TB test, trying my best to weave this all between client appointments as I continued to try to make a living.

With most tests completed, I went for my consultation with the transplant team. My sister Carol came with me. We were both interested in learning if she could be a living donor and thereby remove the need to wait for a compatible liver from a deceased donor. I was incredibly grateful for her support, as it might mean that I could forego the anti-rejection meds, which were known to increase the odds of getting lymphoma, of all things. Because I'd already had it twice, the odds were much higher for me.

Everywhere I turned it seemed there was an extra complication or unexpected twist to my medical conundrum. The assessing physician called us into an examining room and spent the first forty-five minutes interviewing both of us in depth. I was starting to get impatient, frustrated with having to repeat the same old story to yet another physician but realized it was part of his due diligence to ensure we were both amply aware of the risks involved. Carol found the process more interesting as she had not heard it all before.

Finally, the transplant physician closed his notebook and quite abruptly offered a very quick prognosis:

"Well, in our view, you are not ready for a transplant."

As a rationale, he offered, "The odds of you dying from liver disease in the next year are less than the odds of you dying from complications of a transplant. Until it crosses the other way, you will not be put on the list here in BC. Given the condition of your liver, other provinces or the U.S. would put you on a list, but then it would be a long waiting period. Here, we expedite cases when the need arises, which in our view is a more efficient way of matching donors with recipients at the time of urgent requirement."

We pressed the transplant doctor to see if things would be different if Carol was a living donor. He said that it could possibly accelerate things when the time came, but they would not put me on the waiting list for the surgery either way until I was in much worse condition. However, he did encourage Carol to get a DNA test to ensure compatibility if the living donor option was deemed to be a viable possibility when the time came. We thought this amusing as there had always been some doubt whether we were actually identical twins, and the DNA test would confirm that once and for all.

The doctor dismissed us and suggested I come back in six months, or, "or if things get much worse." What, exactly, did "much worse" mean, I wondered. Just as I was mulling this over, the transplant doctor dropped another little lead balloon:

"We are also going to send you for more tests," he said. "We are not satisfied that your cancer is gone. If it is still active, you would not be eligible for transplant surgery." He did not say the words "at all" but I understood what he meant.

The Transplant team scheduled me for an MRI to investigate this possibility. I was horrified that they thought I still might have cancer but thought the MRI would be good way to rule it out.

It only hurts when I breathe

As part of the series of work-ups for the Transplant Centre, I was due the next day for a respiratory consult to look at the results of my recent X-ray and Pulmonary Function Test. When I arrived, my X-ray was displayed in the doctor's office. "Goodness", I said, "that person only has a lung and a half."

"That person is you," he said. "Half of your right lung is compromised by pleural fluid. Do you have any trouble breathing?"

"Understatement of the century," I said. He went on to suggest that I have the pleural fluid drained so they can test it and to make me more comfortable. It was a quick procedure which he scheduled immediately. He met me in Emergency an hour later, and I was grateful for his efficiency.

I drove myself home to make dinner before Rob and the kids got home, hoping to still be able to get to my backlog of client work that evening.

About an hour later, I was in neutropenic shock. My temperature had spiked to 104F, and I was chilled and shaking. I called 711 – the nurses' consult line – only to be told what I already knew: I must go BACK to Emergency, immediately. Rob took me in, an all too familiar routine by now..I was checked in to stay overnight while they flushed me with antibiotics. Halfway through the night I was transferred up to a ward, with a sick sense of déjà vu. The novelty of this scene had definitely worn off.

The doctor arrived the next morning, checked me out and advised that he had no explanation for the infection.

I went for an ERCP scope the next week, and probably would have balked at yet another medical intervention, but this was one I really was familiar with by now. Same old routine, same nurses, old hat. I insisted on the meds, and the procedure happened very efficiently while I enjoyed a light catnap until the doctor came to my gurney-side. Still blurry from the sedation, I had trouble concentrating on what he was telling me. But I came to in a hurry when he mentioned the word "lymphoma". What?? I gleaned the gist of the story: he thought he had seen some nodules – not just a thickening – but was unable to get down far enough to do a biopsy. He was now recommending a "capsule endoscopy" to investigate further.

Were we *really* back in the hunt for cancer? Apparently the only way to confirm this was through another intrusive procedure.

Swallow! You're on candid camera

The capsule endoscopy was quite an adventure. It was actually an interesting procedure designed to take pictures of your gastrointestinal tract from top to bottom; much more effective than silly probing scopes that just don't quite reach far enough down (or up, as the case may be). The objective was to get a good look at the trouble spot in my small intestine. I had to fast for two days. Just what I needed, more weight loss.

The capsule was, in fact, a camera. Yes, after all else I had been through, I was now being asked to swallow a mini camcorder. This little flashing device would record its journey from my gullet to sphincter, sending images by radio transmission to the recording device on my left hip, assuming the battery pack on my right hip did its job.

Fascinating, I thought. The doctor also seemed quite enamored with this technology, describing the quality of the images he would download later this evening. "Great," I said, "may I have a copy on DVD? I'd like to post it on YouTube."

Ultimately, the swallowed camera did its job very well – I have the colour photos to prove it. They are rather interesting if you are at all curious about the secret inside life of the colon. Best of all, the movie version of my innards had a happy ending: my docs concluded that there was NO cancer.

What I had, apparently, was a painfully swollen bowel, probably the result of chemotherapy damage. The condition was exacerbated by foods containing any fat, salt, fibre or certain spices. I was to avoid eating pretty much everything we had in our fridge or cupboards.

In addition to the inflamed bowel, the doctors had identified that my gallbladder had been infected. The various scopes had conveniently cleaned out the infection, but the gallbladder itself was now in very rough shape and would have to be removed. I found myself headed for surgery again.

Normally, having one's gallbladder removed is a fairly routine procedure. But there was nothing routine about my precarious situation. In the latter stages of cirrhosis, the liver cleverly surrounds itself with blood vessels to bypass its inability to do its job. This tends to enmesh the gallbladder in an unpredictable weave of vital veins and arteries, posing a bleeding threat for any form of surgery. In short, it was a very high risk, intricate surgical challenge, demanding an extraordinary skill to avoid nicking a blood vessel. Because I was now under the watchful eye of the BC Transplant team, I learned I was to have the privilege of being operated on by one of the top transplant surgeons in Canada. It was just a matter of when it could be scheduled.

12

A CLOSE ENCOUNTER

E-mail update to my friends and family:

February 2008

No cancer! ... That's the good news. And it is really good news!

And the other news is that they found portal vein thrombosis (blockage of main blood vessel leading out of liver, caused by my liver condition). This would make it too dangerous to have a transplant, so I am now on anticoagulants to try to clear it up. But the anticoagulant treatment could cause a rupture of the enlarged blood vessels in my esophagus, which are also caused by the liver. In addition, I have gallstones, cholangitis (infection of the bile ducts) and chronic edema of the lower intestine (swollen bowel – caused by liver). Very painful. So, basically, I have multiple conditions causing a royal pain in the ass.

In the short term, my gallbladder needs to be taken out, which they tell me is also a potentially danger-ous procedure given the status of my liver.

Wish me luck!

Gallbladder surgery is not viewed as high priority, so the earliest date my surgeon could book was several months away. The surgeon and the doctor were both worried that the infection would flare up again, which would not only be painful, it could be life-threatening. They advised me to go directly to the ER if I had another gall bladder attack, which might enable me to move into the queue for "emergency surgery," given my precarious position.

Not exactly routine surgery

The surgery was finally scheduled. Off I went, quite happily expecting a welcome cure to my current set of gastric discomforts after an easy procedure and a short recovery period. I was scheduled to run a two-day strategic planning conference in three weeks. Throughout my medical journey I had been highly successful at choreographing the timing of my client work around my various appointments and procedures. This was a matter of necessity: if I didn't work, I didn't get paid, and I had no short- or long-term disability insurance to rely on. I had tried to continue with a near full-time workload despite my rapidly deteriorating physical state, finding creative ways of working from home, working from the couch and working from my hospital bed as need be.

I had expected this procedure to follow the same rules. I had completed most of the content work for the conference just prior to my admission to hospital, and I had allotted the week required to recover from the procedure before doing the final preparations to facilitate the event.

But during the procedure, due to my compromised state, I started to hemorrhage. The doctors had to quickly abandon the laparoscopy and do full surgery. I awoke with a 7-inch incision, feeling like I had been hit by a truck. My recovery period would be much longer than originally estimated. Stubbornly, I clung to the idea that I could convalesce quickly. Conor's high school graduation ceremony was scheduled for the following weekend, and I was determined to be there. And of course I was committed to facilitating my client's workshop, which was now just two weeks away. I would have to call on all of my angels to help me to heal as fast as humanly possible.

A week later I was still unable to sit, stand or walk for any length of time. Tragically, I had to admit it would be impossible for me to attend Conor's graduation. I was barely able to get dressed and fix my hair for a few feeble family photos before he had to leave for his proud moment in the spotlight. The photos show a hollow-eyed, scrawny but proud mom, hugging my beautiful firstborn son who is looking suddenly more adult than teen. Conor and I shared some humourous moments hamming it up for the camera until the laughing hurt too much. I posed painfully for more photos with Maddie and Rob, and then off they all went, leaving me wishing sadly that I was well enough to go.

Resting on the couch later, I was the proudest Mom in West Vancouver when friends texted me and sent photos from the graduation ceremony to let me know Conor had won not one, but two scholarship awards for community service.

Ten days later, just in time, I recovered enough strength and determination to run my client's workshop. It was at a resort location requiring a fairly long drive, and I decided at the last minute to take Maddie with me to help in fetching and carrying. It was a brilliant decision. Not only did I get to enjoy her company while working on a fun project, but she also proved herself to be a valuable assistant, even serving as photographer. Her photos were the highlight of the wrap-up slide show for the workshop. After the conference, the two of us extended our stay to indulge in a pedicure and lunch before hitting the road home.

What doesn't kill you

I went for my post-surgery visit upon our return. The surgeon was very forthcoming about his concern about my portal vein thrombosis and my unruly blood vessels. Bluntly, he said I was not a good candidate for further surgery – i.e. a transplant. The fact that I had nearly bled to death during a less complicated procedure was not a good indicator. He also reconfirmed that I was not a good candidate for a living donor situation; he felt I needed more than a partial liver to replace faulty ducts and the portal vein. Ironically, of course, the DNA test had confirmed that Carol was a perfect donor match; there was a 99.98% certainty that we were identical. But, the Transplant Team was not willing to entertain this as a viable option. They refused to put two lives at risk when one was already so precarious.

All of this was somewhat moot, as the state of my liver and related symptoms *still* did not warrant putting me on the waiting list! The Transplant Team agreed it was just a matter of time until I would get there, but my remarkable recovery from the gallbladder surgery was testimony in their view to the fact that I was still healthy. I wondered how it could possibly make any sense at all to wait until I was so sick I couldn't recover from surgery, before putting me on the waiting list for more surgery? Of course, I understood that the surgery could kill me, hence the doctors thought it better to let me keep on living until they needed to pull the final trigger in the game of Russian Roulette that had become my life.

I vowed to redouble my efforts to use complementary healing approaches to defy the odds. I would continue to heal my liver to the best of my ability using meditation, visualization, nutrition, exercise, and my continued spiritual work. I decided that the longer I was able to fortify myself and postpone the need for surgery, the better.

13

CHECKING IN ... OR CHECKING OUT?

"Last thing I remember, I was
Running for the door
I had to find the passage back
To the place I was before

Relax, said the night man,
We are programmed to receive.
You can check out any time you like,
But you can never leave!

—Hotel California, Eagles
Glen Frey, lyrics, 1977

In December of 2008, I belligerently ignored my doctors' advice to avoid salt, fat, fibre and sugar to willfully enjoy the one side-benefit of my condition – my inability to gain any weight. I overindulged in the seasonal cornucopia of cheese dips, ham, turkey, gravy, plum pudding, shortbread cookies, butter tarts – whatever presented itself. I quickly paid the price.

By our anniversary on December 27th, I was packing about twenty-five pounds in extra water around my middle and suffering intense gastric discomfort. I stubbornly insisted on keeping our annual commitment to a getaway weekend at a local hotel to celebrate our twenty-five years of marriage, despite Rob's misgivings. I packed my most forgiving festive clothing, and we enjoyed a wonderful romantic weekend, even though I felt eight months pregnant and could not eat more than a few bites of our anniversary dinner. By the end of our stay I could not breathe while lying in bed; I had to be propped up with pillows. I had trouble getting in and out of the car.

After a few more days, it became obvious my situation was not improving. We decided Rob should take me to Emergency to get my pleural fluid drained despite the fact that it was New Year's weekend. Our timing was terrible, as we arrived at the hospital in the middle of a record snowfall. The triage area was full of portly middle-aged men with chest pains, suffering from extraordinary shoveling activity. Ironic, I thought, as I'd had the same worry about the decidedly unportly Rob, my valiant shovel prince, who had spent most of that day doing hard labour on our treacherous driveway. I insisted that he leave me there and go home to soak his tired muscles, promising to call him in a few hours after the procedure was done. We both thought I'd be home by morning, if not sooner.

However, to my frustration, the ER doc insisted on grilling me in depth, seemingly with the intent of re-diagnosing me from square one. Perhaps he was wondering if I was delusional, because after about an hour of hearing my story, he decided to run a barrage of tests. After all, despite my portly belly, I still did not look like a two-time cancer survivor suffering from end stage liver disease. He embarked on the usual series: blood, urine, ECG, vitals, all repeats of tests I'd had done no more than a month previously in the same hospital. I could not believe this doctor required a fresh battery of assessments just to verify that I should have my now-routine drainage procedure.

Thank heaven he did. When the test results came through, the ER doc advised me that I would be staying overnight as I was in a precarious state. Apparently, in addition to the usual elevated liver enzymes, my kidneys were threatening to shut down, my ammonia was creeping up again and my albumen was depleted.

My visit to the ward of no return

Unfortunately, there were no rooms available. But then the good news came from the nurse that they had found a room for me on the 7th Floor. I remembered that was the Neurological ward, but then she corrected me. "It's on the other side of the floor," she said, "in Palliative Care."

When the time came to transport me, I chatted nervously to the nice gentleman who wheeled my gurney. He seemed to sense my rising panic as we approached the doors to Palliative Care. I wondered if he thought I was dying. Irrationally, I worried that I might actually be left here forever, in the medical version of the Hotel California: "You can check out any time you like, but you can never leave ..."

My nurse was still preparing my bed. How would I explain to my roommates that I was just passing through, not passing on? Would they find that a painful thought and banish me to my own form of purgatory, shut out of their other-worldly clique? Should I pretend I was one of them?

Such wryly macabre thoughts plagued my psyche in the wee hours until I banished them and tried to look forward to this unexpected detour. Maybe I could view it as another stop on the soul train, an opportunity to learn new perspectives. And besides, I would only be here for one night.

But my overnight hope turned into a ten-day exile from the land of the living, a poignant and transformational preview of what it could be like to really be knocking at heaven's door. I now look back on this visit as a gift, a special experience that allowed me to ring in the New Year with some dear souls who knew it would be their last. How lucky I was to still be able to cling to the hope of recovering, with the knowledge that I was only an accidental tourist in this ward of no return.

I settled in to observe my surroundings and assess the lay of the land. In the next bed was Rosie, who I learned had end stage cancer. She had also contracted a hospital superbug, so I could not see her because of the quarantine tent around her bed. However, I could not avoid overhearing her conversations. I was quickly swept up in her unfolding drama.

Rosie was a colourful and gregarious character, still very much engaged in the business of living. By listening to her conversations, I guessed her to be in her fifties. She had many friends and relatives who came to visit, and when they were not in the room she was on the telephone with one or another of them, making plans and sharing news. As the days passed and I continued as a vicarious participant in her various dialogues, I found myself admiring her daily persistence as she cheerily went on with her business. I learned that she was writing a book and marveled at her detailed instructions to one of her friends on how to edit and market the manuscript on her behalf.

One day, her physician came to visit. My curtains were closed. The doctor did not bother to check to see if anyone was eavesdropping as he dispensed with the chitchat in favour of letting Rosie know where things stood. I could not help but overhear as he said in a gentle but fairly clinical way: "I have reviewed the test results. You need to prepare yourself. I think we are looking at two weeks."

By the sound of her gasp it was clear Rosie had not been expecting this. Neither had I. To me, it did not seem plausible, given her current alert state. *Why oh why would he be so finite?* I wondered. I realized it was prudent for doctors to offer some kind of indication, in order to allow people to take the time to put things in order. But I wanted to believe that someone in Rosie's situation could defy the odds, that with her obvious positive outlook and spirit she could possibly push two weeks to two months, maybe a year, maybe more....

But the doctor did not offer her any such glimmer of hope. The "two weeks" he had offered seemed very, very finite. "I thought I had a lot longer," said Rosie with a rasp in her voice. Her words hung in the silence as the doctor left. I was surprised to find I was crying, and I had not yet even seen this woman.

I sat for a while, the invisible witness, wondering if I should remain silent and pretend I was not there. I heard Rosie sobbing quietly. I did not know what to do, but felt it was not my business as an anonymous stranger to offer external support at that moment; I was certain she would reach out to her many loved ones when she had had time to process the news. I curbed my impulse to "help" and decided to respect her privacy. I tried to watch TV as Rosie's hospital stall remained uncharacteristically quiet. But I could not dismiss what I had just heard. I spent the afternoon dwelling on it, almost as if it had been my own diagnosis.

The Rosie who finally emerged was a marvel of purpose. She snapped into the business of preparing her affairs, summoning her mother, sisters and friend to assist with detailed instructions on where to find things, extra keys, the manuscript instructions, computer codes, banking information, pets and so on. It was a sad lesson in what must be done to meet the demands of an event I had not previously had to think about with such a clear focus. I felt quite privileged to have Rosie as a role model in this final rite of passage.

Rosie hung in there for the remaining week of my impromptu visit. I got to know her "in person" when the nurses finally peeled back her isolation curtain. I discovered a surprisingly robust-looking woman about my own age. Her hair was close-cropped, a style I recognized from my own chemo-coif era. Ironically, her super bug had cleared up but she was not ambulatory. I did what I could to help her by fetching things from the kitchen, reading to her or calling the nurse when she needed more morphine. We had some good chats about writing, and I expressed my admiration that she had a completed manuscript. She gave me a few pointers (get a good editor!), and I marveled at her genuine curiosity about my interests when she clearly had more serious things to think about.

Finally, I was given the okay to leave, to return to the land of the living. I will never forget the poignant, knowing look in Rosie's eye as she waved me a cheery goodbye and wished me well. I did not know what to say except, "Take care, Rosie. You are an inspiration."

I returned to the ward to drop off a thank you gift for my nurses just a week later and found to my great sorrow that Rosie had already passed. In the end, she had not even had the promised two weeks. I was deeply saddened at the shock of seeing someone else in her bed. What a privilege it had been to bear witness to the dignity of her last days.

Putting my affairs in order

Until that fateful hospital stay, I had been valiantly trying to continue to work between visits to the hospital. I had been able to manage my coaching and consulting projects around the intense demands of my medical project. But my Palliative Care encounter made me face up to the fact that this was truly a life-or-death situation. It was time to put my affairs in order.

Whether or not the outcome of my situation would be happy, I knew I would be out of commission for some length of time. I wanted to make sure others around me were prepared. I wanted to put my personal affairs into a state I would be proud to leave behind, for a few weeks, or for longer. I decided to take a leave of absence from my volunteer activities.

The next decision was harder: I started tapering off client work and saying no to new assignments. Having spent two years developing my client base, this was very, very painful! Fortunately I was able to call on some trusted colleagues to replace my skills on the more important ongoing projects.

Many of my clients were truly surprised I was at this stage on my health journey, because I still seemed relatively healthy when they saw me (on the good days!). I was proud of that, but realized I had not been doing myself any real favours by pretending things were normal. Once I admitted my vulnerability, I found it actually deepened the bonds of trust with my clients. I was finally able to release some of my fear that my illness would be seen as a failure.

Admit me, please!

By March of that year, the transplant team finally deemed me eligible to be waitlisted for a liver. This felt like a breakthrough, but it also felt scary because of the high risk involved with the surgery. I became an official card-carrying member of The Transplant Waiting List. One of the requirements of remaining eligible was that I needed to have the signed commitment of a caregiver willing to be with me twenty-four hours a day after the transplant. We were not in a position financially for Rob to take several months off work, so I thought of my friend and neighbour Sarah who was currently not working and whose kids were all away at school. Her husband was travelling back and forth to a job in Alberta; hence I speculated that she might have the time to be available to be on-call if she was needed.

I intended only to ask her to help me organize the shifts of friends and neighbours who would share the burden of my caregiving, not to take on the whole responsibility of providing coverage when Rob was not home. I expected to be able to set up the schedule of shifts and dinners in advance, hopefully making Sarah's job easier when the time came. Nonetheless, I worried about the magnitude of the request I was making. It was a lot to ask of anyone.

I needn't have worried; Sarah readily accepted and jumped in with both feet to take charge of the situation. We sent out an email message asking for volunteers and were blessed with an overwhelming response. We had the schedule of shifts set up in no time, including deliveries of pot luck meals to start for Rob and the kids when I was admitted for surgery. Sarah ensured people knew our dietary preferences and best time for delivery, and looked after all of the little details that made it feel seamless for us.

Things were organized on our end and ready for the call, but the transplant system was not holding up its end. After four months of "active waiting", my patience was wearing extremely thin. I learned that British Columbia was experiencing the worst organ donation shortage in the past seven years. No one was able to speculate when a liver might become available.

Despite my frustration, I tried to continue to live as if my life was not hanging in the balance, waiting for life-or-death surgery. Some days I was able to put on such a brave front that I felt like an impostor, so healthy and normal that I almost felt guilty about being on the list. But on the days when my symptoms were at their worst, I found it hard to get out of bed. On those days, I felt like I was in jeopardy of being one of the thirty per cent of people who die while on the waiting list for a transplant.

In late July, despite my fatigue, we decided to have Rob's siblings over for a barbecue party on our deck. We loved these summer Sunday evening deck parties, despite the amount of work involved. We loved to set things up as if we were preparing our home to be featured in *Western Living* magazine. Rob set up the deck furniture and umbrellas while I spent the whole day preparing an extensive buffet of barbecued salmon, steaks, summer salads and other seasonal delights. It was a labour of love, but it left me totally exhausted.

The evening was truly enjoyable despite my fatigue. Our guests left satiated and happy, and Rob kindly did almost all of the clean up after I collapsed into bed. The next day, Maddie arose to find me sleeping outside with my head down on the patio table, still in my nightgown, oblivious to the scorching noon day sun. Rob had left early to go golfing, and Conor was at work. Maddie assumed I was just extra tired, and advised me she was going downtown with friends. I apparently responded in a fairly normal fashion, and off she went.

Following her departure, I finally felt the heat and retired to the couch to sleep, ignoring the remaining kitchen mess from the night before and abandoning any thought of normal routine. I was vaguely aware that I had been sleeping for a very long time, and was still in my nightgown when Rob came home around 3 p.m. In a dangerous replay of my previous ammonia episode, I greeted him with incoherent alarm. He knew the drill. In fact, he had already suspected something was wrong, as he had tried to reach me by phone all day long from the golf course. When I cleared my voice mail several days later, I discovered eighteen progressively more concerned phone messages, one after every hole.

Back in the ER, afraid I would have to re-establish my situation yet again, I asked the ER physician to call the Transplant Team to validate my treatment. That was probably one of the smartest things I did. The ER doc was fairly adamant that I was in very poor condition, and after a lengthy conversation, I learned that I had been elevated to first on the waiting list for my blood type. I was not sure if it was coincidental, or whether the ER doc's call had tipped the balance, but suddenly it felt like wheels were in motion.

This was good news, but frightening because it meant that everyone now agreed that my liver was careening towards failure. The ER docs were once again able to stabilize my ammonia levels, and I was released to the custody of my family, who were warned to watch vigilantly for additional signs of encephalopathy. I spent the next few weeks having to reassure everyone about eighteen times a day that I was conscious and coherent. Every time I made a funny look or attempted humour, Conor repeated his now-favourite line, "Do we need to call someone"?

Meanwhile, we waited for someone to call us.

14

An Alignment of Miracles

....

During this period I was not able to work very actively, nor to function normally. I had been advised not to drive due to fatigue; I did not have the energy to do housework or to descend the stairs to my home office.

While in this state of suspended activity, I sent an update to about two hundred friends and supporters to avoid the speculation and whispers. I had been feeling out of control of my "PR", which is unlike me. Some folks were not aware of my deteriorating state and offered business-as-usual invitations which I could not summon the energy to even answer. Others were worried I was dying, and rather than intrude, discreetly asked friends about my status. I would hear about their inquiry second hand, which was always nice but left me wondering if people were suspecting the worst. I also had to find a way to notify my clients that I would be taking a leave of absence when I got "the call". I decided to use my marketing background to write a detailed e-mail update to everyone I knew.

At the same time, I thought it would be a good idea to try to channel peoples' interest in my well-being to perhaps effect some good in the world by using the message to promote organ donation. It seemed unbelievable to me that people had to wait six months or more for a viable organ, and that a third of the people on the waiting list in BC actually didn't make it. This was partly because at that time, only fourteen per cent of the population had registered as organ donors. Yet registering as a donor is such a simple act, and can actually turn a very sad event into a miracle – by saving up to twelve lives!

Despite having one foot in the grave, I hoped I could still use the other to kick start some change.

August 7, 2009:

Dear Family & Friends:

This is an update for folks who have been kindly tracking my progress through a long health journey. I am entering the final leg of my medical triathlon, as I await a liver transplant. I have risen to the top of the type A blood list (always the overachiever)! I have been advised to avoid going out in public, both to conserve my deteriorating energy, but more importantly to avoid exposure to infections which could make me ineligible for surgery. Basically, I am to cut off human contact for a while.

As someone who loves to go out and meet with folks, this is rather challenging. But, given I've been waiting four months already, with no livers whatsoever being available, I would not want to miss that one alignment of the stars by contracting a tiny virus or cold.

They call the transplant list the "active waiting" list. But I know that's an oxymoron; how does one "actively wait"? If I knew, I'd get right on it. Instead, I'm focusing on savoring every moment by not being active and not frenetically pushing myself in many directions. It seems my

A personality type matches my blood type, but I am now learning to be a B – less doing and more being. That is a whole new reality for me.

I consider myself one of the luckier folks in this state; some people are so ill at this stage that they don't have a choice about being active. So, I am happy to protect my declining health as a shut-in, winding down my work assignments by phone and email, and arranging back-up for my clients to cover my two-month post-surgery recovery period whenever it comes. Tragically, I now look forward to my only outings: I go to the hospital three to four times a week for medical procedures to deal with complications. Hospitals are the ultimate 'no communication zone' – no cell phones, so active waiting is the reality there. I now understand why they call us "patients".

In fact, this waiting game ensures that I actually have time for yoga and maintaining my mind, body and spiritual strength for the journey ahead. I spent the weekend in ER last week unexpectedly (it was air conditioned – could be worse), and even found a corner there to do my yoga. One of the nurses said that I was the healthiest person in liver failure they had ever seen. Hopefully that means my recovery from the invasive surgery will be easier.

My family and I are starting to go stir-crazy waiting for that one special call. The reality is, there has not been a liver available since early March, which is the longest shortage they've had in seven years. It is rumoured that the ambulance strike may be causing some of this because donors are not arriving at hospital on life support. Also, with the resource and time pressures in the hospitals, patients and family are not always being asked about organ donation at time of death.

Ironically, given that I have an identical twin, I could be eligible for a living donor transplant (partial liver). Livers regenerate well so both of us could grow a whole new liver from half of hers. However, the BC Transplant team feels I need 'more liver' than that and it would also put two lives in jeopardy vs. just one. That is a very good point. God forbid I should survive but lose my very special sister in the process.

At one point it looked like the Mayo Clinic in Rochester may have had a second opinion on the living donor option for me, but it would not be covered by BC Medical and could go upwards of two hundred thousand dollars U.S. including travel and accommodation. But even to explore this could mean losing my place in line here in BC, which would be devastating if Mayo ended up having the same opinion as the BC team. I would then be back to square one on the BC list, after an additional delay of a month or more.

No, I will just wait for the BC system where I know and trust my talented doctors. I know the system is still very effective when it kicks into high gear, and will organize itself when it has an organ to offer. I will welcome the services of one of the best transplant surgical teams in North America when the time does come.

Sorry to go on. A friend calls this "the organ recital" and we all know some of those are pretty boring. So, if you no longer find my journey interesting (or never did), just reply with unsubscribe and I will take you off my list. This applies for health updates only, unless you specify no further contact of any kind. That will require a more detailed rationale, however. I promise the next update will be really short: "she lived happily ever after". In the meantime, in lieu of cards or flowers, please just send affirmative thoughts. I'm not great at returning phone calls these days (the former phone queen) but email works just fine and I can use BB in hospital if you want to chat.

Take care of all of your parts, and encourage donorship please! www.transplant.bc.org

—Kathy McLaughlin

After pressing SEND on this message, I spent the rest of the morning cleaning house, doing the same kind of compulsive sorting, labeling and packaging I did before giving birth. But this time there was additional method to my sorting: I wanted to be sure my affairs were in order in case I did not come back from surgery. I knew the odds were not in my favour, and I would not have wanted my family to have to deal with the sad reality of my various piles of work-in-progress.

In my forensic rummaging, I came across a handkerchief given to me a week or two earlier by my friend Sharon. She had called me one day to say she was also having some health challenges, and was going to attend a Catholic prayer mass. She asked me if I wanted her to add my name to the prayer list. I thought this was a very thoughtful call, and a wonderful gesture, even though I am not Catholic. I still needed all the help I could get! To me God is

God, wherever one finds him, so I readily accepted her offer. I even thought for a minute that I would go with her, but I really was not well enough to do that. So I offered her my own prayers for her situation, and off she went.

The next day she brought me a memento of the service: the handkerchief, blessed by the nun's tears. She let me know that the nuns at this Charismatic service had prayed quite fervently on my behalf. I tucked the handkerchief into my lingerie drawer for safekeeping.

Now, several weeks later, I rediscovered the hankie and wondered if it needed to be closer to me to work its magic. I decided it would not hurt, so I tucked it in my bra and went about the rest of my day.

About an hour later I went to check for any responses to my email, and received a premature CONGRATULATIONS message from an enthusiastic supporter who had misunderstood my missive and thought I was already in the hospital getting my transplant. I laughed out loud at that one and said, "I wish!"

At around 7 p.m., I was sitting with Maddie and Rob at our kitchen table having dinner. A helicopter flew low overhead and Rob proclaimed, "There goes Mom's liver!" We all laughed.

Ask and ye shall receive

Then, as if the whole day had been building toward this outcome, at 9:30 p.m. the phone rang.

"Mrs. McLaughlin?"

"Yes?"

"This is Andrea from BC Transplant. We have a donor liver for you. Can you be at Vancouver General Hospital by 11:30 p.m. this evening?"

"Yes, of course," I said quietly, and hung up, turning to Rob and Maddie with tears in my eyes.

It had been about twelve hours since my email send-out. I should have thought of a mail campaign earlier, I joked to myself. As far as direct marketing campaigns go, the response rate had been fairly high – a significant number of recipients had responded to say they had immediately registered as organ donors. I realize it is absurd to think there was any correlation with this good deed and the arrival of my liver – like it gave me extra credits with the liver gods or something. Or perhaps I had activated the nuns' prayers by retrieving the sacred handkerchief. Or maybe it was just a series of happy coincidences – but it somehow reassured me that this was the *right* day, and everything would be all right.

We packed up my things. The drive against traffic to Vancouver General reminded both Rob and I of our late night trek to the maternity ward seventeen years ago when Maddie was born. The memory of our happy anticipation of our new baby daughter helped to lighten the reality that this visit posed a much higher risk and would result in a much longer hospital stay.

But when we got to the Emergency desk, we were left to wait for more than an hour. Something felt wrong. Why was no one in a hurry to get me prepped for surgery? Finally, we were ushered into a hospital room. I was asked to strip, scrub down, gown up and drink a disgusting green medicine – apparently an industrial-strength laxative, I would soon discover.

Then we were told, disappointingly, that the surgery would not be happening as planned. We learned that two livers had come available, and the first one had actually been provided to another patient! I was now waiting for the arrival of a second liver, which was not yet in the hospital. Our nurse did not know when we should expect to be called to the operating room, but at the earliest it would be the next day, assuming the second liver was viable. Rob headed home to bed and promised to return the next morning.

Instead of sleeping (which would have been difficult considering the sudden efficacy of the laxative) I hauled out my laptop and wrote several chapters of this book in rapid succession. I wrote as fast as I could, just in case I did not emerge from surgery. I did not want my story to die with me. I also wrote a letter to Rob, to read to the kids in case that happened. I still have that letter and it still makes me cry.

Rob returned around breakfast time, and I was still flying at the keyboard. He slept in a chair while I typed and typed. I wrote for twenty-four hours straight, between bathroom visits. I spent the whole night and most of the next day purging every last vestige of food and waste from my system, while writing everything I had to say. By mid-afternoon I was officially empty, empty, empty and as ready as I could be for whatever came next.

Finally, the nurse advised that my donor liver had arrived and surgery would be that evening. We learned a bit more about why the first liver had gone to another recipient. After we got the call, while we were driving over, a second liver had been identified. The doctors decided that the second liver was a better fit for my needs, so the first liver had gone to another woman who was next on the list. By now, she had had her surgery and was resting comfortably.

We were finally transported down to the operating theatre at 11:30 p.m. I lay quietly awaiting my fate, with Rob sitting beside me, silently squeezing my hand. The nurses came to wheel my gurney into the starkly lit stainless steel room and I said a poignant goodbye to my patient husband. For the first time in my long journey, I honestly did not feel certain I would emerge from that room alive.

15

PLEASE RELEASE ME

The surgery was a whopping thirteen hours. I cannot imagine the stamina that is required to maintain a precise focus for that length of time. I know I could not do any form of close work for half of that time without going for lunch or coffee. I don't think that's part of the surgery protocol.

I woke up with no knowledge or memory of anything after the anesthetic. I was in Intensive Care with a tube down my throat, doped up on pain killers and raring to go home. I found this to be a repeated irony of my post-surgical experiences: you awake with the memory of how things were before the surgery, and it takes time to believe you are incapacitated. I felt strong and healthy, ready to get up and walk home. Nothing hurt except my throat, which was incredibly dry and chafed from the breathing tube. I soon learned the reality was quite different.

The transplant surgeon came to visit. Since I could not ask any questions, all I could discern was that it had been another close encounter with an early demise, characterized once again by massive hemorrhaging.

Lest I lapse into complacency about my survival, I received reminders from hundreds of people by email, cards and Facebook that I was an inspiration to them. It felt odd to be congratulated for something that was truly beyond my doing. It reminded me to be immensely grateful for the conspiracy of miracles that had granted my pardon. I decided I was happy for others to promote me as a poster child for miraculous recovery if it gave people the inspiration to tackle their own life challenges.

I was discharged from ICU and checked into the Transplant Ward at Vancouver General Hospital two days after the surgery, and set about staging a quick recovery. I ate and drank everything I could get my hands on. I asked Rob to bring in my cellphone so I could communicate with the world, after being incommunicado for too long. On day three after surgery I did a walkabout with my physiotherapist and sent a photo to my friend Judy to update my Facebook page. It probably looked like I was showing off for my fans, but in fact I was simply reveling in my ability to walk, talk and function after my incarceration in ICU. My birthday was September 21st and we had every reason to expect that I would be home well before that.

The following day, just when I thought I was out of the woods and well on my way to early discharge, I found myself facing another excruciating struggle. Despite my quick recovery and early mobility, my abdominal pain had continued to escalate. Anyone who has had a caesarian or hysterectomy will agree that abdominal pain can be excruciating. Just as I was coming to terms with that level of pain and thinking it was all I could handle, things spiraled out of control.

Finally, the head of the transplant team came to see me. I thought he was here to help with my pain, but that was not what was on his mind. The day before he had visited to tell me the good news that all of my indicators were going in the right direction. But today, he did not look so cheerful. "Your enzymes are up, which could mean rejection. We will do an ultrasound, and maybe a biopsy, then decide on treatment. If it is rejection, the usual treatment is a mega dose of steroids. That usually works. This happens at some point to many people, so not to worry." But of course, I was worried. The only good news was he authorized some additional pain medication for me.

Over the next few days my liver took hold nicely and showed no further signs of rejection. All of my vital signs were moving in the right direction. I was mobile – able to walk without my walker, fix my own meals, walk up and down stairs, and dress myself. Despite a nagging low-grade temperature that puzzled the nurses, the doctors thought everything was fine and since I had no other symptoms they were preparing to sign my release papers within the week. I was feeling relieved, deeply grateful for my return to good health and eager to resume a normal life.

16

INSTANT REPLAY

As fate would have it, the Gods of Infirmity had not finished with me yet.

My body temperature continued to be a concern, and my blood tests started to reveal a low hemoglobin count. Initially, these symptoms were viewed as normal by-products of transplant surgery. However, one night I attempted to go to the bathroom and collapsed on the floor, too weak to stand. My temperature had spiked to 102F and the night nurse gave me Tylenol and put me back to bed. My morning blood test showed that my hemoglobin count was dangerously low. My doctors were puzzled; there was no evidence of hematoma at the surgery site. Yet I suddenly required a transfusion of two litres of blood.

An ultrasound revealed internal hemorrhaging. The cause was determined to be an internal infection which had been quietly gaining momentum in my abdominal cavity and was now rapidly threatening my new liver. Emergency surgery was required to stop the bleeding and arrest any further damage.

I don't remember much from that point on. In fact, I have no memory of how I got from the Transplant Ward to the operating room, or what happened after that.

Seven days later, I suddenly awoke in a strange room, intubated and completely immobilized. I felt like yet another truck had flattened me; the pain was excruciating. A strange face was smiling at me, a pretty blonde doctor I didn't recognize who was reassuring me that the procedure went very well and they were very proud of me. *What procedure?* I wondered, having no idea how I got here, how much time had gone by or when I might see a familiar face. "Your husband has been here every day," said the pretty doctor. "He is such a lovely man". *Just how many days is she talking about,* I wondered. "Your liver is doing very well so far," said the doctor. *Of course it is,* I think. I have no recollection of the infection or the bleeding; in my mind, I am still focused on going home in a few days. *Why am I being held captive by these strangers?*

Slowly, with utter horror, I realized I had received a **second** transplant. Apparently, during the surgery to assess the bleeding, the surgeons had decided that my new liver had suffered too much damage from the blood loss. They had put me into an induced coma to wait for another liver. I learned, incredulously, that I had lain unconscious in ICU for nearly a week. Finally, my family had been told that if another liver was not found in the next forty-eight hours, it would be too late.

In times such as this, the transplant team broadcasts the need for an organ to all other medical institutions within a forty-eight hour delivery zone of the hospital. This increases the chances of retrieving a suitable organ, but it is still dependent on a random set of circumstances. Essentially, the only thing that could save my life was the loss of another person's life, at the right time, in the right place and in the right way. It is a horrifying thing to have to wish for.

It is quite unbelievable to me that, once again, the universe summoned a series of miracles on my behalf. First, another soul lost his or her life at the appropriate moment, leaving behind their legacy of life, less than 24 hours after the call went out! Second, my doctors decided to take the heroic risk of allocating that precious liver to me, despite the low odds of me surviving another major surgical procedure. Third, during surgery, the doctors yet again had to pull me back from the brink, after my compromised arteries caused massive hemorrhaging. And fourth, my spirit somehow found the superhuman strength to battle back to life after the surgery, though my body had come closer than ever to giving up.

As for me, the only thing I recall from my near-death experience is a dream-like vision where I was out at sea, frantically trying to save myself from drowning. I was swimming for dear life but was totally, utterly spent, exhausted to the point of giving up. Just as I felt like I was slipping further into the deep, I thought about my kids and Rob. Suddenly, I felt a superhuman surge of energy, like a bolt of electricity throughout my whole body. At the same time, I was propelled forward, as if a powerful wave had come to carry me to the shore.

It was not until several months later that Rob was able to tell me his side of the story of my survival. For him, the worst moment of all came when I was in the recovery unit, still comatose and clinging to life after the all-day surgical ordeal. It was late at night and the hospital was quiet. Rob was sitting at my side, and a male nurse came to take some readings from the wall of monitors surrounding my bed. Rob asked the nurse when I might be able to leave the recovery area and go back to my room. The nurse looked alarmed and said, "please stay right here. I'll be right back."

A few minutes later the resident doctor came in to talk to Rob. "Do you have any idea what is going on here?" he asked. "I don't think you realize how serious this is. Your wife is not going anywhere in the very near future. Do you see those dials monitoring her progress? Things are very precarious. She may not make it through the night. Right now, her heart is beating harder than it would be if she was running a marathon. No one can sustain that level of effort for too long. You may want to pray for a miracle, my friend."

And so he did.

Ingrate inmate

But the day I woke up in ICU, I was certain someone had made a serious mistake. As I started to appreciate the full reality of my situation, I became really, really angry. I still can't explain that reaction. It was a little like running the race of your life, seeing the finish line just ahead, and then waking up back at the start line without the use of your arms and legs. Fortunately, I was unable to articulate any of this to the unsuspecting intensive care nurses, as I fear they would have found me incredibly ungrateful for having my life saved.

Partly because of this rude awakening, and partly because I felt so incredibly weak, vulnerable and sick, my time in the ICU felt like sheer torture. It was only a period of ten days or so, but it felt like the movie *Groundhog Day*. Each day was a grueling repetitive ordeal and each minute was an eternity. I would awake from a fitful, short sleep, not knowing if it was morning or evening. There was no clock in my room, no radio, and no evidence of the outside world. I did not know what time it was, what day it was, or what was going on in my family's lives. All I could see out the window was the sky and the top of a building where there were no signs of life. As I gained consciousness, my pain made itself known and each day I discovered a whole new litany of symptoms as my body awakened to its new reality. I started to experience very threatening psychotic dreams. Everyone around me was part of a conspiracy to kill me, or at least to find new and inhuman ways of torturing me.

My fear was exacerbated by my inability to communicate. I was intubated, so unable to talk. It took me a while to become stabilized, both mentally and physically, and I slowly realized what had actually happened to me. Fortunately that coincided with being extubated, and once I could talk my anger and frustration had mostly dissipated, in favour of immense appreciation for what the ICU nurses go through, day in and day out, with disoriented and delusional patients.

I still experience a mixture of intense sadness and gratitude when I think about what my donor and his or her family had to go through for me to be spared. I am guessing many transplant recipients experience this kind of survivor guilt, combined with an overwhelming appreciation for the gift our donors bestowed at the moment of their passing.

17

RE-CONNECTING WITH MY COMMUNITY

I arrived back on the Transplant Ward unable to use my arms, legs or back. I was quadriplegic, the result of three weeks of atrophy and starvation. My return to the ward miraculously coincided with my friend Sarah's return from her summer cottage. She promptly took over managing my communication with the outside world, assisting me at bedside and organizing caregivers for my return home. She came to the hospital nearly every day for several hours, taking turns reading to me, bringing or preparing food to ensure that I ate, putting lotion on my now HUGE feet and legs (water retention from my many intravenous liquids and other drugs) and running intervention when the nurses were busy.

I cannot say enough about the incredible support she provided, as did the network of my relatives and friends she organized to babysit me when I returned home. As one small part of this, she sent out email updates on my behalf, which filled in the blanks when I could not connect with my followers on my own:

Sent: Friday, September 18, 2009 9:16 a.m.

Subject: Kathy M - September 18th Update

Hi everybody

I don't have Kath's wonderful writing skills but I know you all want news, some of which you may already know.

Kathy had a second liver transplant on September 4 after she got a massive infection. She's had a number of surgeries since then to close her up. She clawed her way back and finally got out of intensive care on Wednesday and she was moved back up to the liver transplant ward. Unfortunately, her exit from intensive care was short lived ... she had emergency surgery again last night as she was hemorrhaging again. She's in recovery. It's been quite a journey for her.

Kathy knows that everybody is thinking about her and pulling for her. She doesn't want any visitors, she is concentrating all of her strength on recovering and she doesn't want the risk of exposure to any germs/infections.

I will be in touch just as soon as I know if there is something you can do for her or the family. At some point we hope to be able to launch the "caregiving plan", but we're not there yet.

Sarah

Sent: Friday, September 18, 2009 6:29 p.m.

Subject: Kathy M – September 18th Further Update

Hi again all

I just spoke to Kathy and I wanted to convey to everybody that she's okay after last night's surgery. She says the surgery seems to have patched up what needed to be patched up (not exactly her words!) and she is back on the liver transplant ward. She hopes to send her own e-mail update to you sometime in the next few days.

She was pleased to hear of everybody's good wishes.

Sarah

Sent: Thursday, September 24, 2009 5:11 p.m.

Subject: Re: Kathy M - September 18th Update

Hi All

Greetings from Kathy and she thanks you all for your positive thoughts and good wishes. She feels she is definitely back in the land of the living, and the family and I all concur. The light grows brighter at the end of the tunnel.

We celebrated Kath's closing ceremony today with Thomas Haas pastries; she had a nibble of several of them. The closing means that last night marked the last of her surgeries (...we hope). She has now been entirely stitched up with a new liver inside. Some of the side effects of the medications are anxiety, depression and mood swings and she seems to be running through a full gamut of those, but those are temporary. Over the next couple of months, medications will be fine-tuned and she will be restored to the same old (whoops young) Kathy that we have all come to know and love. She's on a liquid diet for a day or two and then back to solid foods, which she is very much looking forward to.

Kathy has of course plugged herself back into her cell phone. If you speak with her you may find she sounds a bit dopey as she is still on pain medication. She is also still recovering from the effects of having had a tube down her throat for a while; but I can assure you she is all there.

She hopes to be home in no time, but it's going to be a slow and gentle recovery process as they don't want her to tear any of her very delicate insides. The hospital will still be her temporary home for a while longer, but I'll keep you posted as her recovery progresses.

Kathy longs to be back at work and doing a multitude of other things!

No visitors please (except immediate family). It's not that she doesn't want to see each and every one of you, but she's not up to it. She continues to focus all of her energy and strength on her recovery.

Sarah

Sent: Tuesday, October 06, 2009 7:11 p.m.

Subject: Kathy M - Update October 6, 2009

Greetings ... Kathy says it's time for another update. She had some wonderful one liners, which I was to incorporate into this e-mail but I wrote them down and then left the pad in the hospital! Hmmm and she's relying on me to make sure she takes her meds on time? There could be problems here ...

Kathy really is progressing. One of her many liver doctors (I can't keep track of who's who, it wasn't a surgeon but somebody else who keeps track of liver function), came in today to tell us that her liver was functioning well according to her most recent tests. So now the focus is on getting her back on her feet (gently), getting rid of the cathe-ter and the bed sores, and encouraging her to eat as she doesn't have much appetite. Physio today went exceptionally well. She is still not allowed to sit or bend at the waist but the physio and nurse got her up today and she was able to stand with a walker and then walk to the end of the bed and back. There is still work to be done on her leg muscles and her breathing but she was congratulated by all today for her fine progress. She's also working with some squishy balls that Rob gave her to get her fingers moving so that she will have an easier time with keyboarding and working her cell phone.

The doctor today thought Kath might be able to go home in a week or two, but that will depend on how she progresses with her physio. There's still a fine balance between pushing the physio and not blowing a gasket in her insides! She needs to be able to get from the house up the stairs to the car and back because I know I'm not going to be able to carry her and I suspect the same goes for Rob. J

Stay tuned ... I think I'm getting closer to requesting help with some caregiving shifts and food
arrangements for when she gets home.

Sarah

Sent: Monday, October 19, 2009 5 p.m.

Subject: Kathy M - Update October 19, 2009

Rob has gone to pick Kathy up and she will be
home this evening. She is going to be exhausted
tonight and tomorrow as it's been a busy day visiting the transplant clinic, the physiotherapist and
the occupational therapist. But all medical staff are
supportive of Kathy's desire to be home.

She won't be running a marathon yet, but she'll be
working on it, one day at a time.

Sarah

When I got home, Sarah had organized two shifts a day of four
hours each, for friends, neighbours and family members to take
turns sitting with me, helping with my meds, helping me to the
bathroom, making tea, reading books, or watching movies together.
This was perhaps the most miraculous time of all for me, in the
sheer delight of connecting with caring friends and loved ones after
the lengthy ordeal I had been through.

Since my second cancer diagnosis, when I visited InspireHealth
and learned that one of the attributes of people who experience
cancer remission was that they "reconnect with their sense of community and reclaim the joy that comes from being of service to
others," I have made a point of connecting with new and old friends.
Whereas the old, work-focused me would have been much more of

a social recluse, I started to readily extend and accept invitations to play bridge, go out for coffee, walk the seawall, have lunch.

The healing power of kindness

It is now overwhelming to think back on the incredible support I received, over and over again, from my many well-wishers. These are people who don't need a wake-up call to get the message to be in service of others. Their profound thoughtfulness was humbling. From gourmet potluck dinners, to incredibly thoughtful gifts, cards, messages, I was truly overwhelmed by the healing outpouring of love I received. Although there is no way I could ever repay their kindness, I resolved to do everything I could to pay it forward, whenever others need that kind of support, or simply empathetic conversation and constructive encouragement.

If I had one piece of advice for anyone in life, it would be to reach out, be connected, find the joy in learning what's in peoples' hearts. Have coffee, lunch, phone conversations, send email – don't hunker down and wonder why no one calls you. This is not a contest to see how many people will come to your funeral; it is an appeal to enjoy the love that this life can provide, so you can postpone your funeral. Especially when you are trying to heal from a life-threatening illness, it is time to reach out and connect with those you would miss, or those you would regret not having gotten to know better.

For me, each caregiver shift was a gift of connection, a chance to get caught up on peoples' family news, hopes, fears, frustrations. I learned how to get past my well-developed walls to engage in authentic, heart to heart conversations – okay, with maybe a little gossip sprinkled in. I had fun watching old movies in the daytime with no guilt, crying and laughing with my kind friend Helaine, who seemed to know just the right ones to pick. We both looked forward to our "Tuesday Morning Pajama Parties".

Each person in their own way provided just what I needed: a hot cup of tea, quiet time for a nap, gatekeeper phone answering, or assistance to walk to the bathroom and stand sentry while I did my business all by myself, thank you.

Those who drove me to the Transplant Clinic and doctor visits gave the physical gift of loading my wheelchair, learning to navigate backwards down our precarious driveway, which I could not even begin to negotiate; and supporting me up the stone steps to the car.

The gift of getting to know my parents

I also got to know both of my parents much more intimately during my recovery period. Dad had come to the hospital every three days, bringing me home-cooked meals that were exactly what I needed. He was nearly eighty, hard of hearing, and slightly forgetful, so I am certain these trips were a bit of an ordeal for him; not to mention the difficulties in preparing a meal for me with his painfully arthritic hands. When he came, we would sit and talk for at least an hour. Several times I read him the passages in my journal describing my memories of childhood. He listened intently, and we would have conversations about how he saw things. At one point he said, "I had no idea you thought so deeply about these things." It was the first time in our lives that we had talked in such depth beyond the "how are the kids / what's wrong with the world / how's work" level of banalities, and those had usually been in a family get-together where one-to-one chats were rare.

Similarly, Mom and I had become much closer even before I was admitted for the initial transplant. She had taken me shopping, or our favourite excursion: heading to the beach during the glorious summer that preceded my hospital stay. We both bobbed about in the surf at Spanish Banks like beached whales. In my then-bloated state it was a delicious relief to cool down and lose gravity for a while in the relatively clean and truly refreshing ocean water. We had long chats about the universe, her beliefs, her regrets, and our mutual medical complaints. We seemed to have similar ailments at similar times, including aching feet, midriff bloat, shortness of breath, etc. Never mind there were twenty-five years between us; it was hard to tell who was healthier, but my guess was her. We had always been able to talk about more profound matters, but in my previous busy-work state I had often been dismissive of what I felt was her "belief of the month". I now realize there is a beautiful pattern to her search, in her consistency of knowing there is a universal energy, be it interplanetary life or other forms of wisdom. Some of her theories are too "out there" for me, but I have learned to listen and often learn from her search.

I can only view both of my parents now with a deep compassion for being who they are, and a profoundly better understanding of them.

The fourth InspireHealth attribute of patients who heal is: they bring a new authenticity to their relationships with others and the world around them. I did not consciously set about to do this; it was simply what happened when I allowed myself to slow down and take the time to receive.

18

Happily Ever After?

"Life is a gift, and I try to respond with grace and courtesy."

– Maya Angelou

As I write, more than 5 years have passed since my second transplant. Those are years I would not have enjoyed without the gift of my new liver. I knew I had been spared by a series of miracles, and that I could find a new purpose in that reality. Yet my first year "back" was extremely difficult both mentally and physically.

Physically, I had to undergo intense physiotherapy to regain the use of my arms and legs. The ordeal of back-to-back transplants and nearly four months in hospital had caused my muscles to atrophy. I wondered if I would ever enjoy a normal life, even a walk on the seawall without feeling fatigued. But, slowly yet surely, I built strength and started to resume many of the activities I thought I had left behind. By January I was able to travel and we took the kids to Hawaii. It was Maddie's last year in high school, and Conor was attending university. They both readily sacrificed their studies to enjoy a week in the sun. I scared the heck out of the whole family by partaking in a Sea Doo adventure which nearly shook my new liver loose. I was determined to enjoy every moment and every adventure to the fullest extent possible.

But lurking in the background was a new threat I did not expect. Behind the poignant joy of survival, I was fighting off a growing sense of bleakness. I knew I should not squander the new life I had been granted; but I had no conviction about what I should be doing with it. Every time I thought about the life ahead of me, I became incredibly weary. I was 54 years old and I had no real job. Our financial situation was challenging, due to the market declines and my lack of income for several years. Our kids were almost grown and would be leaving home soon. My parents were getting old. I felt like I had missed the best years of my life, and everything that lay ahead was hard and sad.

By the early Spring I was consumed by an overwhelming sadness. All I could think about was what I had lost, and what losses lay ahead for me. Maddie was in Grade 12, and every soccer game, every drive to school, every family dinner, every lunch I packed reminded me it would be the last time. I had already missed so much of the kids' lives, working and battling my illnesses. Everywhere I turned the people I loved and things I enjoyed were being taken away.

Why had I been robbed? Why had I been spared to now endure this tragic reality? I had received a miraculous gift and all I could think about was that I did not want to be here. I knew how ungrateful that seemed, which made it all that much harder to articulate to anyone. Everyone around me was so glad for me - how could I tell them I was not glad to have survived? I had been abandoned by my positive compass, the one thing that had always been there to pull me through. In many ways, this was worse than any ordeal I had yet faced.

I now recognize how insidious depression can be. It tricks you into thinking your negative thinking is sound. It robs you of the motivation to fight back. I did realize this sad, despondent person was not me, and I desperately wanted to have me back. But at the time I felt powerless. I had no certainty that I would ever recover my previous "pathological optimist" persona. I seriously wondered if my personality had been changed forever; maybe my new liver had brought alien DNA into my system, which had invaded my psyche. Throughout my physical ordeal I had relied heavily on the power of my positive will to help me navigate. To be robbed of this faculty seemed the cruelest joke of all.

As my dark thoughts got darker, I realized this was not normal. I started to read about post-traumatic stress disorder, which I had previously only associated with war and horrific accidents. I learned to my surprise that it is not unusual for PTSD to occur after a traumatic illness.

I mustered the motivation to see my GP. Choking back tears, I described my state of mind. The doctor confirmed that I appeared to be suffering from a form of trauma-induced depression that was treatable. I was immensely relieved to learn this was not simply my new state of being. Finally I had some hope that, with treatment, I could rediscover my enthusiasm for life. The GP referred me to a psychiatrist who prescribed antidepressants and gave me a referral to a mental health program. Just the realization that I was in the grip of an illness was somewhat reassuring in getting through it.

As relieved as I was, for the first time in my long health history I felt terribly sorry for myself. How unfair was it to be sick, again, and to be robbed of the one faculty that could help me shake it, the positive outlook that had seen me through all of my prior challenges? How ironic is *that*?? I felt like a helpless victim, most of all because I could not find a way to tell anyone how I was feeling, even those closest to me. I tried to act normal when the kids and Rob were around, but spent my time alone crying and sleeping.

I only took the anti-depressant medication for a week because it made me lethargic and stupid, which in fact made me feel worse about myself. I did, however, attend the mental health program, which consisted of weekly group therapy. After others in the circle had talked about their problems and suicidal thoughts, it was my time to tell my story. The first time I told it, it sounded miraculous and inspiring to everyone but me. People sat looking at me in stunned disbelief of what I had lived through. One girl burst into tears and said it was the most inspiring story she had ever heard. I was certain they all wondered why I was there, HOW I could possibly be depressed when I had been blessed by a series of miracles.

Each week we were asked to give an update on how things had gone for us and what thoughts we were having. After a few weeks I started to take some joy from giving others a source of inspiration for at least an hour a week.

I also bought some audio tapes on ways to beat depression, and started to push myself to exercise a little bit each day. Everything I did helped a bit, but ultimately time was the best healer. It took another six months for me to feel fully reunited with my optimistic self.

Back to Life

As I write this, more than five years later, I often feel as if this whole story is about someone else. The dark places I have been are so at odds with the joy I find now in everyday life. I am working full time as a management consultant and have built my business back up to a very rewarding enterprise. I am striving to save something for our retirement, while also embracing opportunities to travel and indulge in the best life has to offer, including travel with my family, social time with friends, volunteer work and quiet personal time. I play tennis three or four times a week, and work out at the gym. I am working hard, most days, but with the satisfaction that comes from doing work I love and having an impact on those I work for. I enjoy the perfect balance of work and play and I love the clients I choose to work with.

Smiling back at the old "work-first" me, I now remind myself to make time for family first. I am involved in my kids' lives and as supportive of their launching careers as they want me to be. My parents are healthy mid-80 year olds, and I see them often. My sister instituted weekly Friday lunches at the iconic White Spot Restaurant with Mom, an occasion that includes any grandkids that happen to be around. When I once complained about always having to go to White Spot (which Mom loves), my wise sister said "think how much you'll miss it when she's gone". So I look forward to it, every week, and invite my kids whenever they can make it.

Finally, I am able to look back on my ordeal with the blessing of objectivity, and look forward to the future with a renewed optimism. I have had time to reflect on what messages I can take from all I have endured on this extraordinary journey. I feel I owe it to my readers who have endured along with me, to share that learning.

Stuff happens

I have learned that we cannot rely one hundred per cent on the medical experts. As talented as any individual may be, the system is such that mistakes can happen.

I have learned that when mistakes happen, there is no upside in laying blame. I encountered no acts of negligence; just the harsh realities of a system that is sometimes dysfunctional. My medical team were all well-meaning, smart people who did the best they could. There is a lot of judgment and sometimes luck involved in the outcomes of decisions and procedures.

I have learned that the patient can provide a great deal of the variable input to lower the risk and increase the odds of good luck. It also gives you a stronger sense of confidence in the outcome when you are involved in the decision-making and make yourself part of the team. As InspireHealth points out, people who recover from terminal illness "regain a sense of control in their lives – a feeling that they can substantially impact their own health and healing. They assume responsibility for creating a recovery program that is right for them - they do not simply abdicate responsibility for their treatment to their doctor."

I have learned that assuming responsibility does NOT mean throwing your weight around and demanding results. It is a collaborative process, and sometimes your doctors will hear you out and provide reasons why your suggested approach is not recommended. At least you get the reasons, and sometimes you may cause them to rethink their first judgment call, which is all good.

The body's just the start

I have learned that healing from illness is not just about healing the body. It is an invitation to heal at a deeper level of mind and soul. That is a journey I am still on and indeed it is a life-long, daily practice that is just part of who I am. It consists of living each day with immense gratitude, practicing heart-based communication with others, and continually aligning my actions with my purpose. Reminding myself to "speak only what heals". Again, this is one of the attributes of cancer-healers identified by InspireHealth: "They undergo a 'spiritual transformation' – an awakening of the true values and aspirations that had lain dormant inside them. Truly alive – perhaps for the first time – this spiritual re-awakening brings a new authenticity to their life as they reconnect with their deepest values and aspirations. Once healed, they may look back upon their illness as a 'gift' that helped transform their life."

I have learned that work is not life. My work now is an expression of my soul. I put myself in the service of others and try to use my experience, knowledge and skills to meet their needs, often more profoundly than they had hoped. As I continue to align myself in this work, somehow I receive clients who are on the same wavelength, and we almost always become friends in the process. I used to draw a severe and permanent line between my work and social life: never the twain shall meet. Then I spent so much time at work I had no social life. Yes, I was trying to avoid something, or at least to ignore it. That something was my heart. I never let it out to play.

I have learned that now is the time to express my voice, without worrying about what others think. This does not mean judging, blaming or criticizing others. It means bringing authenticity and integrity to my communication, to speak only healing words. Sometimes that means sharing the story of a miracle. I have been privileged to be able to do this in my many talks about my experience. One of the moments of which I am proudest was when I was asked to be the keynote speaker at the BC Cancer Foundation's Inspiration Gala in October 2010. I was honoured to be invited to talk about my experience with lymphoma. The talk was meant to be only five minutes. I was scared stiff despite numerous rehearsals. When my name was finally called I stood shakily at the podium, staring into the floodlights and the sea of five hundred faces representing Vancouver's most influential VIPs. I realized these were just people like me, each of them touched in some way by cancer, here to support others suffering from this insidious disease.

I spoke from the heart, told my story, and expressed my gratitude for the outcome of my journey. I was astounded to receive a standing ovation, and more astounded to learn I had talked for twice my allotted time. People were crying, cheering and applauding. At the end of the night, the Foundation had raised $1.3 million more than their goal. I felt proud of my contribution to that and so grateful for my ability to use my story to give something back to the medical community who had helped me through my journey.

Expect miracles

"There are two kinds of people: those who look for miracles and find them, and those who don't look for miracles, and see none" - C.S. Lewis, *Miracles*, 1947

I have learned to be wide open to see the little miracles that occur every day. Whether they are truly miracles, or just predictable coincidences that I choose to see as miracles, they are happy little events that make my heart sing. They point to the synchronicity, the pattern, the flow of this mysterious thing called life. I encourage everyone to see their own miracles. If you don't believe me, start by invoking the parking angel. I have taught many people this trick. Next time you are rushing to get somewhere, call on the parking angel just before your arrival. Unfailingly, she will come to your aid if you are open enough to see that spot.

I have learned that living "happily ever after" means fully embracing the gift I have been given of a renewed chance at life. It means living in every moment, recognizing that the journey is the reward, and there is no "someday" – it is now. Being fully present enables me to see the abundance around me and bring all of myself to the party. It means bringing the whole me – all of my creativity and energy – to every encounter. It means asking the question "how can I serve" at every opportunity, from the note I write in a greeting card, to my daughter's need for homework help, to my mother's call to chat. It means casting aside judgment and irritation for exuberant acceptance of what comes next. Loving what is.

And I learned powerful lessons about how I was choosing to live my life. Instead of driving, working, rushing and blaming, I learned to STOP. It finally dawned on me how many of life's moments I had missed by being absent, sometimes physically, but very often mentally as I thought about plans, schemes, next steps and how to achieve more. As this became clear, I realized I had to develop an entirely new skill; I had to learn to be present for what was left of my life.

Take a pill and chill

To change my approach I had to stop paying lip service to 'being' and seriously go cold turkey on 'doing'. I had to learn to relax, agree, accept rather than take up arms at every slight frustration. I had to keep my weapons (my anger, ego, intellect and caustic humour) at bay long enough to listen to my heart. In the corporate vernacular, I learned to "pick the hills I wanted to die on" and choose only the battles that were profoundly important, based on true life priorities. After all, how important was it, really, to stay late to write a blistering email to the finance department for shortchanging my operating budget by three per cent, when the other choice would have been to go home to enjoy dinner with my family?

By opening my heart and seeing others' behaviour as well-intended, I learned to convert acrimonious gun-battles into rewarding human exchanges. I also learned to convert my going-in stance of critical distrust to a more trusting and accepting attitude. By finding my way to this zone of compassion and forgiveness, I found I could tap into the miraculous ability we each have to embrace life, *now* – with our mind, body and soul.

It means operating from a fundamental starting point: love. Not fear, not anger, not superiority or the ego-protective warrior stance. Just love. It is so much easier.

19

Taking Control

....

*4 first steps that helped me on
the path back to wellness*

If you or a loved one has recently been diagnosed with a life-threatening illness, here are 4 keys steps to set you on the right path as you begin your journey to wellness.

*Step one: The most important
homework you'll ever do*

Thank goodness for the Internet. There is no longer any excuse for a patient not to be extremely well informed about their situation. The big challenge is filtering the facts from the fiction, and the hacks from the experts. As I did my deep dive into everything written about cancer in general, Hodgkin's Lymphoma, autoimmune liver disorders, and any evidence of the two running concurrently in other patients, I started to learn which websites to trust, and which to avoid.

My best advice is to read everything, and you'll start to see the patterns in recurrent information. You will also start to recognize by the dates and sources to determine whether information is old, questionable, or contradicts the generally accepted data. Such sites as

The Mayo Clinic, www.mayoclinic.com, Medhelp, www.medhelp.
com and sometimes Wikipedia (with caution) are excellent to give
you an overall scope of your illness, a particular procedure, etc.
You can Google almost anything by name - chemotherapy drugs,
medical procedures, treatments, doctors' names and treatment
records, to get the information you need.

What is the information you need? In my case, I wanted to know
all about the various treatment options for my two life-threatening
conditions. I read everything I could find in the reputable medical
journals and sites detailing treatments, side effects and trials. Then
I read about alternative and complementary therapies such as
acupuncture, yoga, Qi Gong, meditation, reflexology, supplements,
exercise, diet and psychotherapy. For most of my life I had shied
away from new age-y, holistic or alternative treatments that touted
themselves as "miracle cures".

But as I explored the latest sites and blogs, I started to realize
there were some important developments in what is now called
"complementary" care. I read with excitement about the science of
integrated healing, which advocates choosing a treatment regimen
that includes complementary therapies in partnership with the
medical system, to enhance the healing process. To me, this seemed
to offer the best of both worlds: ancient wisdom drawing on the
intrinsic abilities of mind, body and spirit to self-heal, combined
with the best medical science had to offer. At the stage when my
medical team was pretty much baffled about what to do with me,
I found some hope in the idea that I could do some of my own
work to move in a healing direction. Rather than surrender to the
thought expressed by one of my specialists that "there is nothing
we can do", I chose not to include myself in that particular "we".

This gave me the preparation I felt I needed to make some
informed choices about my treatment plan. I knew I wanted to
include things I could do for myself to support the good work of
my conventional medical practitioners. At this stage, I didn't know

which complementary therapies I would apply, but I knew I wanted to allow space in my plan to do more research in this area.

If I had not done this preliminary homework, I know I would not be here writing this book today. I would have been totally reliant on my medical doctors for my treatment plan, and two things could have happened. First, I might have bought into their perspective that my situation was hopeless. Second, I would not have been able to fortify my body so that it could survive chemotherapy, fight my cancer and support my ailing liver.

Meanwhile, to be positive about who's in charge, the first step is to do your homework. Read everything. Ask your friends and relatives to read everything if you don't have the energy. On my worst days when I didn't feel like getting out of bed, I downloaded audio books and podcasts to my iPod so I could read between dozing. At least I felt like I was doing something positive instead of feeling sorry for myself.

Step Two: Creating your own healing roadmap

Drawing on my corporate training, I knew the next step after researching the situation was to set some goals for my project. In context with the bleak prognosis I was getting from my doctors, this was somewhat like setting a "big hairy audacious goal" (BHAG) - the term business gurus use to get corporate teams to focus on a daunting task.

The key to goal setting is to start with a vision of where you will be 5 to 10 years from now, and then establish mini-goals along the way to track towards the vision. The vision can be "aspirational" - something bold and wide in scope like "to lead the world in widget-making". In the context of my health challenge, the 10-year goal was pretty clear: "to be here". However, the real key to setting a BHAG is to think outside the box, even beyond what is possible, to make it truly exciting. So, I decided to go for it "all": my BHAG for 10 years from that point was:

"I will be embracing life, in exceptional health, excelling in my career, with a healthy, happy family, loving marriage and rewarding friendships."

By sitting down and writing this out, I was able to get myself out of the mind-set of thinking I was "sick" - end of story. All of a sudden I was focused on the whole me, the rest of my life beyond my disease, and how I could keep moving on all aspects of "me" beyond my illness. This gave me the inspiration to keep looking ahead.

From there, it was a simple matter of defining the milestones to get there. This is the part where I had to pretend I was really in charge. It may seem preposterous, but I actually wrote out a project plan:

Project: Heal Kathy McLaughlin
Goal: Achieve complete cancer remission with minimal side effects, and restore liver to full functionality in the next 12 months.
Action Plan:

1. Assemble team: ensure the right people on the bus

   a. Get a second opinion on cancer diagnosis - ASAP (KMc)

   b. Get a second opinion on liver condition - ASAP (KMc)

3. Complete diagnostic phase by end of First Quarter 2005 (ONC, GI)

4. Enroll in integrated health workshops - ASAP (KMc)

5. Fortify liver to withstand chemo by end of First Quarter 2005 (GI, KMc)

6. Determine cancer treatment plan and schedule (concurrent – by end of Second Quarter 2005) (ONC)

7. Execute cancer treatment plan to achieve a minimum 80% reduction in malignant mass by end of Fourth

Quarter; full remission by end of First Quarter
2006 (ONC)

8.   Minimize damage to liver, lungs, kidneys, etc. (All)

To me, there has always been something miraculous about writing out a set of goals "as if" I had control of the situation. It may be easier in a corporate setting when you are the boss and people pretty much have to do what you say. But even there, it is hard to get people to follow along unless you can convince yourself that you are in control of the situation and act from a position of confidence in the outcome. Sometimes it requires turning off the part of your brain that wants to enumerate the many reasons why things can't be done, or won't succeed, or haven't been tried before. I have found it a lot easier to press the OFF button on those objections when I have a written plan in front of me with deliverables, dates and assigned responsibilities.

I did not actually share the plan in this form with my doctors. But it enabled me to interact with them from a foundation of positive confidence, with a direction in mind.

I encourage you to write down a plan, even if you don't feel like you are in charge of the situation. If you don't have the energy to write, dictate it to a friend. When I was at my worst, I asked my Mom to type up my handwritten notes. She was delighted to help (she LOVES to type) and she was ecstatic to be involved in my plan. We both felt less helpless because we were taking positive steps towards being in charge.

Step Three: Assemble a positive team

When your GP first suspects cancer, liver disease or any other "special" condition, he will refer you to a specialist or two. He is usually guessing about your illness, and also working within his own frame of reference about who are the best specialists in that area.

This does not always mean you will get the best expert, or the right expert, to diagnose your illness and recommend treatment.

I have seen many patients in the medical care system who are not happy with their doctors. To me, this is like making a bad hire. It is your responsibility to do something about it. Either learn to respect and appreciate your doctor, or fire him or her and get a new one! I am not sure why people assume they have to take the doctor they are given.

To verify my cancer diagnosis, my GP sent me to an oncologist associated with the local hospital. He was a very efficient, matter-of-fact, experienced professional. He seemed quite certain about my treatment, the outcome and the side effects. But an element of uncertainty was introduced when he asked me to participate in a clinical trial offering two alternate courses of treatment. The trial involved a random draw, and when I was selected for one particular treatment, my doctor made it clear he favoured the alternative treatment, which was more aggressive but had fewer long term side-effects. I tended to agree with him based on everything I had already read about both treatments, but we agreed it was a good idea to get a second opinion. The second oncologist recommended the conservative treatment – the one I had been selected for in the trial.

Many people might have surrendered to the experts at this stage, but I was not satisfied. My oncologist and my research had planted seeds of doubt about the long-term side effects of the conservative treatment. I decided to seek a *third* opinion, from another local oncologist whom many friends and neighbours had recommended. Though it was somewhat unconventional to get a third opinion, my doctor agreed to give me the referral. For me, it was the only way of obtaining reassurance.

The third doctor's opinion was to opt for the aggressive chemo-therapy-only treatment. This oncologist explained that in his view, I was too young to take the risk of having bladder or organ cancer later in life as a possible by-product of the radiation. "If you were 20 years older, perhaps, but we want you to have a good long life," he said, with a kindly pat on the shoulder. I was consumed by gratitude for this compassionate man. It was at that point that I decided, not only would I choose the aggressive treatment, I would switch to this oncologist for my treatment.

You ARE in charge of who's on your team. It may sound presumptuous, but I firmly believe you need to choose who you will work with when you are fighting for your life.

Using headhunting skills to recruit your team

I know that assembling the right medical team was a critical factor in my survival. My health challenge was so complicated that at various times I needed an oncologist, gastroenterologist, hepatologist, radiologist, respirologist, surgeon ... and that was just on the medical side of things. I wanted to be sure that my roadmap included complementary therapies, so I also needed to find a variety of other practitioners to support my plan: a yoga instructor, acupuncturist, nutritionist, reflexologist, chiropractor and naturopath. No matter what type of professional I was looking for, I followed the same process to find people I trusted, who had a good track record. I employed the same techniques I learned in my executive recruiting career.

Identify your "candidate pool"

When being referred to a specialist by a GP, people often think they must accept the first choice they are given. But I have learned to ask my GP to offer me several choices, and to tell me what he knows about each one. This may not always be possible if there is only one specialist in your area, but in larger metropolitan areas there are usually several choices. Although some doctors are reluctant to critique their colleagues, you will still be able to gain some good insights from your GP about the track record and reputation of the people he refers. You and your doctor can make an informed decision based on his best information. Or, you can take his suggestions away with you and let him know you'll get back to him once you've decided who to see.

There are many places you can go to get information about doctors or other professionals. I asked my friends, my medical team, even people I met in hospital waiting rooms, who they were using in each of the areas I wanted to explore. As I got to know the medical office assistants (MOAs) in each of my doctors' offices, I realized they were a wealth of information. There were several occasions when an MOA gave me some insight on a surgeon or other specialist's interpersonal skills and helped to steer me away from a bad choice.

You can also do online research to find out about a professional's reputation. It is surprising what you can learn by Googling a doctor or practitioner's name. There are sites such as *ratemds.com* that provide very useful reviews by other patients. As with any internet research, you must be selective about what you take from the information presented, but you can find some extremely helpful perspectives based on other peoples' experiences.

The initial interview

Once you've decided which doctor or professional you will be seeing, your work is not done. The first appointment is very important in your decision-making process. I like to refer to this as "the initial interview". I say this with some humour, because most doctors don't act as if they are applying for the job of being your doctor. Quite the contrary; I have had some initial meetings with specialists where I felt like I was the one being grilled. That is why I found it critical to arrive fully prepared, with a list of well-researched questions, a notepad and pen.

I learned over time that it was also important to take a "positive partner" with me to help. When there were two people in the room, both asking intelligent questions, I found doctors took me more seriously. My partners were usually my husband – dressed in his business suit; or my sister, a provincial court judge. While this was not calculated on my part, I have no doubt in retrospect that having one of these two well-dressed professionals in the room helped to establish an air of mutual respect, adding to my confidence that I was in charge of the situation.

Whoever you take, you need to be certain that person is positive and professional. I recommend that you both dress nicely so that the doctor feels like you respect him. Just as you are there to "interview" your doctor, he is also forming an impression of you. I also recommend that you avoid taking anyone who is overly emotional, negative or frightened. As much as I love my Mom, I had to stop taking her to my appointments because she wanted to blame the doctor for my many side effects. I appreciated her concern on my behalf, but I realized that these normal side effects were outside of the doctor's control and her complaints would only serve to alienate him.

With your positive partner in tow, armed with a list of well-researched questions, you are now in a position to assess whether this is the right doctor for you. By asking your questions, you should be able to get a reading on whether this is someone you can work with, collaborate with and confide in as you go through your healing journey. You will also signal to your doctor that you want to be fully informed and involved in decisions regarding your treatment. Many doctors respond well to patients they view as responsibly involved in their treatment decisions. In fact, many prefer that to the alternative; a passive "victim" who does not take the time to educate themselves on the details of their diagnosis and treatment program.

I found there were a few times when I decided not to work with a particular practitioner after the first appointment because he or she did not have time for my questions, or somehow made me feel like my questions were dumb. But most times, I got the answers I needed and established a positive footing for our future interactions.

Step four: Your healing bible: how keeping your own records can save your life

Being positive about who's in charge also means that you need to be on top of your own documentation. I found that as I was referred for each new procedure or consult, the technicians I encountered had remarkably little information about my situation. Sometimes I would show up for an appointment and be sent away because my lab reports or x-rays had not yet arrived, or historical records had not been sent over by the referring physician. I am not a patient person, and I quickly became frustrated with the game of "hide the health record".

I realized that I would have to be the point person for data collection so that I could carry "the whole story" with me to each appointment. I set up a binder with separate sections for my own notes from medical visits; blood tests; technicians' reports after each procedure; surgeons' reports and hospital records; and background information such as drug monographs and patient instructions.

The dilemma was, how do you get your hands on your own documentation to do this? I found there were two answers to this question at the time; and now there are three. The first was to ask each doctor to write "copy to patient" at the top of any lab requisition (blood tests, x-rays, scans). This does not always work and not all physicians are willing to do this, but it is always worth asking. The second answer was to fill out a requisition to the Patient Records department of each hospital I attended. The first time I did this I requested all of the information they had back to my original cancer diagnosis. It took about four months to get the data and it was a two-inch stack of paper! It was fascinating reading and I quickly learned which reports were useful and which were redundant, so that the next time I requisitioned my records I was more selective in my choices. I got in the habit of updating my binder every few months, and with smaller requests the information arrived more quickly.

The third answer arrived after my recovery, with the recent advent of online lab test results - hallelujah! I am now a proud subscriber to BC's My eHealth service, which provides access to my monthly blood test results within about 24 hours of collection - well before they are needed for any upcoming appointment. Many areas now offer this kind of online tracking of medical tests.

Be positive about who's in charge

The important thing to remember is, you are in charge. If you take responsibility for doing your up-front research, creating your healing roadmap, selecting your team and keeping your own records, you will set a positive leadership model for your healing journey ahead. Others will have no choice but to follow.

ACKNOWLEDGEMENTS:

The folks who saved my life:

I must first acknowledge Dr. Paul Klimo. I am so grateful every time I see this lovely man in the mall, on the seawall or out driving his distinctive car – which seems to be every few months – all I can say is thank you for persisting and sharing my faith until the miracle did happen.

I would not have been here to write this book if it weren't for the diligent good care and incredibly wise counsel of Dr. John W. Zohrab, partnered with his trusty sidekick, Medical Office Assistant Barbara Buchols. From the day I was late for my first appointment with Dr. Z, through to the day years later when I bumped into him in an elevator with his post-retirement golf tan, I have thanked my lucky stars that he studied my case and sleuthed through the muck to find some answers to my dilemma.

Similarly, my two transplant surgeons, Dr. Charles Scudamore and Dr. Andrezej Buczkowski skillfully navigated the maze of my portal venous system not once, or twice, but dozens of times before their job was done. I slept through most of that. The fact that they offered me a second chance to get it right, despite the odds and the poor job I did of keeping the first liver, was quite miraculous and I am grateful to them every day.

I can't say enough about the donors of my two livers. To think that *two* thoughtful souls lost their lives, and in the process gave me the gift of a new lease on life, is such a profound thought that I am still in awe. Such a simple decision, made at a time when they were healthy, probably living busy lives, but not too busy to register as organ donors. I send thank you notes through the BC Transplant clinic to their families every few years on the anniversary of my transplant, even though I have no idea who they are. I tell them I am living the best life I can, every day, in honour of their loved one's gift.

My angel friends

To Sarah James, who took about two seconds to say "yes" when I asked her to take on the role of back-up caregiver after I got home from my transplant ordeal. Originally I asked her to fill in on the days when Rob was at work. But in typical Sarah fashion, she proceeded to dispatch her responsibilities pretty much 24/7, with the cheerful, confident competence of a professional. So much so that my Dad thought she was the nurse-in-charge at the hospital, and in fact she did seem to know more than anyone about what was going on at any given time. Sarah: thank you for the foot massages, conversation, clean underwear and magazines; for renting and picking up the Red Cross equipment, schlepping my wheel chair up and down our narrow front steps, and arranging the dozens of shifts of friends and family to bring food and sit with me.

Thank you to all of those friends and family who visited, brought food, gifts and cards, movies and games, read books to me, helped me to the bathroom and up the stairs to the car, drove me to doctor's appointments, updated my Facebook page – the list of kindnesses goes on. I will never be able to repay everyone, but I hope to be able to pay it forward whenever anyone in our community needs me for anything.

My family

They say that serious illness is always harder on the family members than it is on the patient. I know in Rob's case this was definitely true. I can't think about his incredible support without melting into tears. How he endured the long hours of uncertainty and the many inquiries of "how's Kathy?" while keeping up a chipper daily routine for the kids, I will never know. So many times I awoke in the quiet early morning darkness of my hospital room to see him standing beside my bed, a silent and shadowy sentry until he saw me open my eyes and greeted me with a cheery "good morning beautiful!"

To my Mom who wore her worry as visibly as she wore the yellow gown and nasty rubber gloves each time she came to visit in the hospital. Who brought me candies and books, happy stories of what was going on outside in the real world (or on TV), and kept up the brave, positive front every time I was re-admitted to the hospital. I am truly sorry for the dark cloud that must have haunted you while I was in such a precarious state, and I can only hope I will be there for you whenever you need me as we enjoy our remaining years together.

To my Dad who braved impossible traffic, frustrating parking lots, hospital germs and doctor phobia to visit me regularly with lovingly made pasta, Alaskan cod and roast chicken, despite his arthritic hands. Thank you for sitting with me and listening as I read chapters from the manuscript of this book and giving me, as always, your keen take on my verbose sentences. Life is too short for long sentences. I'm still learning that.

To my sis, Carol, the robust twin, who always found ways to carve time out of her incredibly busy commitments in service of others to join me for medical appointments, and in her matter of fact way always asked all the right questions to get answers and results. And while I was in the hospital, thank you for repeatedly and cheerfully responding to my imperious pleas for urgently-required popsicles, or a list of truly unnecessary necessities (the steroids made me rather demanding, as you still remind me). You are my role model for living life to the fullest while sharing your gifts with the world.

To Andy, for always being there with your wit and humour, especially when you visited in the hospital and blew up the rubber glove. I laughed so hard I almost gave back the liver.

And, last but never, ever least, to Conor and Maddie, my beautiful, supportive, patient, funny, happy, inspiring and soul-nurturing children, for always rolling with the punches and making me feel like I was a normal mom. Even when I was bald, nauseous, fat, skinny, yellow, blue, purple or grey. When I was sad, happy, mad, really mad, hysterical or terrifyingly silent.

To Conor, for the way you worry with a big smile on your face, and the way you make the serious seem tolerable with your quick quips and easy chuckle. For coming with me inquisitively to my first chemo appointment, and for sitting by my hospitable bed in almost every ward in every hospital in Vancouver. You made me so happy when I lay in bed feeling sorry for myself for missing your grad ceremony, but then received dozens of text messages about your proud walk across the stage to accept not one, but *two* scholarships, despite all the setbacks and worries you endured through most of high school. It is both ironic and gratifying that you now work at the hospital where I spent so many days and nights throughout your adolescence. You always make time to help other friends and strangers just when they need a friendly face, and it warms my heart every time I hear of your compassion. It also warms my heart when you call and invite me to taste your latest kitchen creation.

To Maddie, for crying when you found out I would lose my hair, and then gently cutting my patchy strands off with as much style as possible. You helped me immensely with shopping therapy when

I most needed it and wardrobe advice even when I didn't think I needed it. You made me so proud when I came to attend your big fashion show in Toronto. I am in awe of your confident embrace of the world and have been blessed to be welcomed by you as a tag-along companion on parts of your journey. You have encouraged me up so many mountains: the literal ones - Devil's Bridge, Camelback, The Chief, Grouse Grind (nearly), Mount Batur, the mountain temple in Croatia. And figuratively, when I did not think I could conquer the next setback, your cheerful expectation that I was well kept me going. I look forward to climbing many more mountains with you.

My editors

My manuscript went through many edits, but no editor was so effective and brutally honest as my friend and colleague, Leslie Hayden. Thanks to her ruthless blue pen, this book is mercifully shorter, more readable and less likely to land me in court.

I invited numerous volunteer readers to endure chapters and rewrites, and am hugely grateful to every one of them for their welcome encouragement and critique. I am particularly grateful that you endured the loony parts of early drafts and maintained your faith that I would eventually get past the catharsis and throw that stuff out. Thanks to you, parts of the story have been left out to protect the innocent. ☺

And now, back to life.

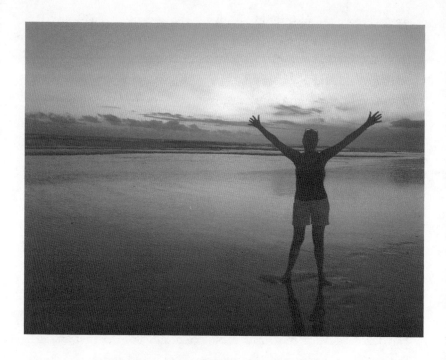

The author, Seminyak Beach, Bali, Indonesia 2014
Madison L. McLaughlin, photographer

ABOUT THE AUTHOR

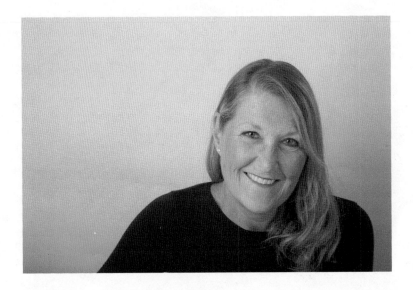

Kathy McLaughlin lives in West Vancouver with her husband and has two grown children. She works as a management consultant, motivational speaker and executive coach. In her spare time she enjoys every waking minute, playing tennis and golf, hiking, kayaking, skiing, cooking, reading, writing, walking, parasailing ... and whatever else life offers up. She is currently working on her second book, a guide to miraculous survival.